Effective
Therapy

EFFECTIVE THERAPY

MICHAEL J. HURD, Ph.D.

Dunhill Publishing Co.
New York

EFFECTIVE THERAPY

A Dunhill Trade Paperback

Published by:
Dunhill Publishing Company
A division of the
Zinn Publishing Group
ZINN COMMUNICATIONS / NEW YORK

ISBN: 0-935016-23-6

Printed in the United States of America

Library of Congress Cataloging-in-Publication Data

Hurd, Michael J., 1963–
Effective therapy / Michael J. Hurd.
p.   cm.
Includes bibliographical references.
ISBN 0-935016-23-6 (pbk. : alk. paper)
1. Psychotherapy.   2. Self-help techniques.   3. Consumer education.   I. Title.
RC480.515.H87 1997
616.89' 14—dc21   97-3285
                                                   CIP

Table of Contents

Acknowledgments

I wish to express sincere appreciation to the following individuals, some living, some dead; some of whom I never met. All helped make this book possible.

To Dunhill Publishing Co., my publisher;

To Benjamin Gill, for his thoughtful and useful revisions;

To Brenda Gressman, for thorough and conscientious editing;

To my parents, Robert H. Hurd, Jr., and Margaret M. Hurd, for encouraging me to read and to educate myself;

To Ayn Rand and her philosophy of Objectivism, whose emphasis on reason and individualism provided both the intellectual and emotional fuel for writing this book, and whose ideas have inspired me to develop a rational approach to psychotherapy;

To Cynthia Sterling, my agent, for recognizing the potential of my manuscript and for successfully finding a publisher;

To Mark Maier and the staff of the Lee Shore Literary Agency for their contributions to this effort;

To the late Clota Yesbek, who understood the importance of intellectual honesty;

Most of all to Bob Yesbek, for his unwavering support, suggestions and inspiration.

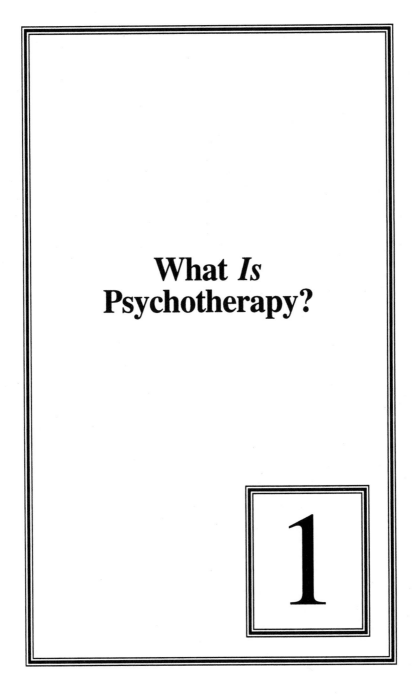

What *Is* Psychotherapy?

1

Psychotherapy is the misunderstood stepchild of American medicine.

Erroneously stereotyped by physicians and the general public alike, it seems remarkable that psychotherapy continues to be in such demand. Despite the enduring images of slick leather couches and eccentric old men with thick accents, it remains the treatment of choice for everything that God, medicine and the government cannot solve.

What *is* psychotherapy? A common sense definition does not yet exist. In fact, many believe that common sense and psychotherapy are mutually exclusive concepts. This book will demonstrate that psychotherapy and common sense *are* compatible, if one approaches the issue in a logical and clearly focused manner. Even if you have had a negative experience with a psychotherapist or psychiatrist, you will learn from reading this book that good therapy—and, more important, the *ideas* underlying good therapy—can be a highly effective tool for improving your life.

In the broadest sense, psychotherapy refers to an alliance between an individual and a mental health professional to seek resolution to an emotional or interpersonal problem. Like all human relationships, the one between therapist and client involves an exchange. Ideally, the client is trading money for the time, expertise and guidance of the therapist. As a return on the investment of his money, the client expects more insight about his problem than he previously possessed and possibly even a resolution of the problem.

The therapy relationship resembles few other human associations. Though both business and professional, it involves more intimate contact (in the nonsexual sense) than any other relationship in one's life. Therapist and client can talk like friends, but the purpose of the session is to discuss the client's personal concerns, not the therapist's. The client also has the opportunity to experience an unusual kind of relationship, whether it lasts for just one session or for several years. The therapist puts constraints on the relationship, such as length of time to talk, availability after hours, fee structure, and so on. A highly unique blend of professionalism and intimacy, of rules and flexibility, characterizes the therapeutic relationship.

Despite the notion of therapist-client relationship, psychotherapy, along with its parent discipline, psychology, is a young science barely making its first steps. Today's psychologists are observing and gathering material from which a future science will emerge.[1] It is a mistake to place psychology on an equal par with physics, chemistry, biology, and neurophysiology. On the other hand, psychology and psychotherapy are not branches of religion or mysticism. Psychology involves the study of cognitive and mental functioning. It uses rational scientific methods to determine the truth or falsehood of its numerous hypotheses and conclusions. Psychotherapy consists of applying psychological principles to the resolution of specific emotional problems.

Although psychology is a distinct science, a variety of professionals comprise today's psychotherapy field, each one claiming a wide array of credentials and subspecialties. A distinction must be made between *objective* credentials and *claimed* credentials. Objective credentials refer to degrees, certificates, or special training which are subject to validation as either true or false. For example, a psychiatrist either has a medical degree, or he does not. The credential is subject to verification or proof, usually in the form of a diploma or license. In terms of objective credentials, three kinds of mental health professionals comprise the marketplace: (1) psychiatrists (physicians with medical training); (2) doctoral level therapists (individuals with a Ph.D. in psychology but without medical training); and (3) therapists with a master's degree (clinical social workers, psychiatric nurses, licensed professional counselors, marriage and family therapists, etc.).

Objective credentials, while very important, should not be the deciding factor in evaluating a potential therapist. The deciding factor depends upon what one is seeking. Only psychiatrists, for example, can prescribe drugs. On the other hand, most non-medical mental health providers have enough knowledge of medication to make a good tentative assessment of whether or not medication is a requirement of treatment. "Psychiatry" generally refers to the medical practice of prescribing mood-altering drugs such as antidepressants. "Psychotherapy" involves the nonmedical technique of talking with clients about their emotional or interpersonal problems. Many psychiatrists do not practice psychotherapy and rely on the doctoral and masters-level clinicians to provide such services.

Claimed credentials refer to the specialties a particular therapist might claim to possess, but which are not easily objectified. A therapist may claim to be a sexual abuse specialist, for example, or an alcoholism specialist. The consumer needs to understand that specialties in the mental health field do not always refer to specific, prolonged training in the specialty area. A hypnosis specialist, for example, did not attend an extra year or two of medical or graduate school in order to acquire his specialty, although he may have participated in a number of professional conferences (which are often brief in duration and do not issue a formal degree).

In my opinion, clients ought to seek a therapist with a good approach based upon a rational philosophy of life rather than one with a particularly exotic or dynamic specialty area. Specialty areas, of course, are useful if they accurately reflect the number of years a therapist has worked with certain types of problems. At the same time, expertise in specialty areas cannot replace competent therapeutic methods. A good approach to therapy teaches clients the proper principles of coping with emotions, and gives them methods for applying these principles to their particular problems. These principles have wide application to a wide variety of individual problems.

Good and bad therapists are to be found among all of the mental health disciplines. The objective credentials tell you something about the therapist, but do not tell you whether a therapist is good or bad. If objective credentials, while important, do not by themselves determine the effectiveness of a therapist, then other criteria are required.

This book has four purposes: first, to identify an objective set of criteria for evaluating a therapist; second, to use these criteria in evaluating the existing models of psychotherapy; third, to describe an alternative approach to therapy in "client-friendly" terms; and, fourth, to consider the wider impact psychotherapy has on society in such areas as parent-child relations, the cost of health care, and the erosion of personal responsibility. Neither the practice of psychotherapy nor its consequences occur in a vacuum. As therapy becomes more popular, recognition of the impact of psychotherapeutic ideas on both the individual client and larger segments of society are essential to the fulfillment of this book's purpose.

"How Do I Solve This Problem?"
The Schools of Psychotherapy

Consider the following example.

Mr. J. thinks he should change jobs, yet he experiences terror at the thought of doing so. He cannot say why, other than that he has a vague feeling that he will not do well on his new job. He has held his job for twenty years. His wife is trying to persuade him to change careers because he does not make enough money, and she feels he deserves a more challenging job. Mr. J. agrees with this reasoning but nevertheless still feels stuck. What should he do?

Now, imagine that Mr. J. seeks out a team of mental health professionals, each with his or her own theoretical approach to psychotherapy. Each of the fictitious psychotherapists on the mental health team represents, in undiluted form, one of the major schools of thought in today's marketplace; "undiluted" because most psychotherapists do not practice any one particular school consistently. Nevertheless, these ideologies, acknowledged or unacknowledged, set the tone for the field of psychotherapy that typical clients encounter each day.

After careful assessment, the clinicians make their recommendations:

Dr. Advil: "I believe that Mr. J. needs an antidepressant. I think that he has a chemical imbalance, and that correcting it will help his low self-confidence and need to please others, which I believe are holding him back in his job. He should remain on this drug for at least a year."

Dr. Erotico: "Mr. J.'s problems all began in childhood. Many of the clues to his problems reside in repressed childhood memories. Although he cannot remember, at one time he wanted to have sex with his mother, and he feared that his father would cut off his penis. Because he never resolved this normal stage of life properly, he has grown into a shy and intimidated man who fears advancement on his job. Unconsciously, he thinks that other men will castrate him for going after what he wants. I recommend a five- to ten-year period of psychoanalysis so that he can resolve these problems by talking with a therapist and having a corrective emotional experience."

Dr. Fido: "Mr. J. was never reinforced for hard work as a child. Consequently, he developed into a lazy adult. The fact that his job does not pay very well has merely reinforced that laziness over the years. Humans essentially resemble animals in the following respect: if rewarded for a behavior, they will do more of it; if punished for a behavior, they will do less of it. I recommend therapy to help Mr. J. expose himself to conditions where he can be more favorably rewarded for what he does. Only then will he be willing to take on a tougher job which pays more."

Dr. Sensitive: "Mr. J. needs more unconditional love in his life. His wife, for example, is making things much worse. Instead of assertively expressing her opinion about his low self-confidence, she should simply say that she loves him for who he is, *with no conditions whatsoever.* She should never criticize him, because criticism is never constructive. Unfortunately, we live in a callous and selfish society in which children are taught to be competitive and judgmental from their earliest days. Mrs. J. and the other individuals in Mr. J.'s life cannot easily overcome this dog-eat-dog mentality, but if they do, he will certainly develop greater self-esteem. All he needs is love."

Dr. Ecology: "Mr. J. is not the problem. Individual psychological problems do not exist. Only *family* pathology exists. Perhaps Mr. J. and his wife have many unspoken marital problems which keep him from advancing. Perhaps he, his wife, and their older daughter constitute a dysfunctional relationship. One thing is certain: the family needs to be cured, not Mr. J."

Dr. Shaman: "I do not see Mr. J.'s current life as his problem. I see his *past* life as the origin of his troubles. Four lifetimes ago, before his present incarnation as Mr. J., he lived as a female in the Middle Ages. His (rather, *her*) lover went off to fight in the Crusades and never returned. The man offering Mr. J. the new job, in this lifetime, is actually that lover in reincarnated form. Mr. J. can't remember any of this but, with hypnosis and past-life regression, I can help him remember it all. How do I know all this? I just do."

Dr. Gloom-and-Doom: "Mr. J., the adult, does not feel vulnerable about tackling the new job; his inner child does. We all have a child inside of us who feels hurt and rejected, and has never recovered from the hurt and rejection in his childhood. All the times he asked his father for help, and his father ignored him; all the times he brought home something from school, and his mother refused to look away from her housework; all that drinking his father did. The inner child needs nurturing, caring, and attention before Mr. J. can expect to do anything else in life. Mr. J. is a victim of forces outside of his control. Healing the inner child will take a long time and involve a great deal of pain and agony. One cannot escape the consequences of a childhood filled with rage, rejection, and utter despair. Mr. J. needs lots and lots of therapy."

Dr. Advil represents the psychiatric (or medical) school. Not all psychiatrists share the medical view. Many psychiatrists, while strong proponents of medication treatment for mental problems, nevertheless agree that psychotherapy is crucial for helping emotionally distressed individuals. Dr. Advil's error lies in his apparent assumption that physiological factors are the *sole* cause of low self-esteem and depressed mood. His decision to treat the client with medication rather than try some form of psychotherapy first follows from his mistaken premise.

Dr. Erotico represents psychodynamic or insight-oriented psychotherapy. Dr. Erotico's diagnosis was inspired by Sigmund Freud's theory of psychosexual development. While Freud did contribute some significant ideas to the young field of psychology, many of his theories were bizarre, contradictory, and arbitrary.[2] Classical psychoanalysts, as doctrinaire followers of Freud are still called, believe that personal change will occur through a *transference* process between the therapist and client. Transference basically means that the client, through an unconscious or uncontrollable process, will project his mother, father, or other important childhood figure onto the therapist, and that the establishment of a long-term therapeutic relationship will somehow result in a cure. Psychoanalysis, despite the many volumes on the subject, is still mystical and anti-scientific because nobody has yet been able to explain it in terms most clients can understand.

Another major problem with the psychoanalytic view is that the cure can take years, and no known objective criteria for measuring the success or failure of such treatment exists. According to Freudian theorists, early childhood experiences shape all of one's adult values, beliefs, and emotions.

Dr. Fido represents the behavioral school of psychotherapy in its undiluted form. Like Freudian theorists, behaviorists subscribe to the theory of *determinism*. In psychology, determinism means that an individual's psychological make-up is the exclusive product of factors outside of his control. Determinism is "the theory that everything that happens in the universe—including every thought, feeling, and action of man—is necessitated by previous factors, so that nothing could ever have happened differently from the way it did, and everything in the future is already pre-set and inevitable. Every aspect of man's life and character, according to this view, is merely a product of factors that are ultimately outside his control."[3]

Behavioral theorists claim that people do not have independent, reasoning minds and that the rewards and punishments of others determine all human action. Individual values, goals, and preferences are irrelevant. The implication is that you, the client, are nothing more than a trained animal responding to stimuli in the environment.

Behaviorism and behavioral therapy became popular in the 1930s, as a reaction to the lack of objectivity in Freud's theory. Behaviorists were concerned that Freudian therapy focused too much on the past and did not provide objective, observable criteria by which to measure treatment success or failure. Their solution, unfortunately, involved ignoring the mind altogether and shifting to an exclusive focus on behaviors. In so doing, they replaced one illogical theory of human nature with another. Behavioral therapy overlooks the view of humans as rational animals with the capacity and necessity for thinking, long-range planning and creating changes in their environment.[4]

Dr. Sensitive, the undiluted version of humanistic (or client-centered) therapy, assumes that a therapy client can be loved into feeling better, with little other effort required. "All you need is love" summarizes the philosophy underlying client-centered therapy. Applied consistently, this philosophy would mean a criminal could be *loved* into goodness; a lazy person could be *loved* into being a hard worker; and an Adolph Hitler could be *loved* into closing his concentration camps without the use of force.

We have not yet loved our way out of poverty, crime, and social unrest. In fact, Dr. Sensitive's popular notion that love is a feeling with no relation to reason has contributed to contemporary social problems such as divorce, unwanted pregnancies and promiscuity. In practice, seeking love without reference to logical judgment leaves one's fortunes in the romantic arena entirely to chance and range-of-the-moment emotions. Humanistic therapists never intended such circumstances to develop, but no other result can occur if the notion of "unconditional love" remains the social and personal ideal.

Humanistic theory and therapy conflict with the rational idea that all genuine love implies some kind of conditions. A mother loves her own child more than a stranger's, because the child is her own. A happily married man loves his own wife more than other women because of the special qualities which attracted him to her. Romantic love and friendship arise, to a significant degree, from the perceived characteristics and values of another individual. Emotions are not causeless. They arise in the context of previously formed conclusions and value judgments. It is impossible to separate the notions of love and value judgments without destroying what is uniquely human about all of us. Unfortunately, the unconditional love premise of humanistic therapy teaches clients the opposite.

Dr. Ecology usually calls himself a family therapist, although he may also call himself a marriage and family counselor, or simply a psychotherapist. The Dr. Ecology form of therapy can create serious problems for clients. Like Freudian and behavioral therapy, it is deterministic. Dr. Ecology's therapy rests on the premise that individuals are molded largely by factors outside of their conscious control, particularly from emotional, physical and sexual abuse in childhood. Some ecological therapists find evidence of abuse in the childhood of virtually everyone, and usually recommend years upon years of expensive therapy and vaguely defined "working through issues" in order to make any progress at all. Instead of teaching victimized people how to become strong and move on with their lives, they encourage clients to adopt the label of "abuse survivor" and endure a prolonged, self-effacing victimization status for a period of years or even a lifetime.

According to the ecological view, most mental health problems arise out of past and current family dynamics. Family dynamics do not simply refer to the various relationships among individual family members. According to this view, there exists a "family dynamic" apart from and other than the mere interaction of individual family members. A family therapist might put it this way: "There is a family reality as well as an individual reality."

Such a statement unnecessarily confuses the issue of family dynamics. Thinking logically about the definition of "family," one can see that the family consists of individuals, each with his own characteristics, viewpoints, and behaviors, who interact with one another in a particular social/biological context. The family does not reside in some separate sphere of reality divorced from the world in which the actual individuals live. If psychological problems do arise, their origins reside in the mistaken assumptions and behaviors of one or more of the individual family members. A mother, for example, may seek to excessively interfere with her daughter's school work because of a mistaken assumption that her child's grades are indicators of her success or failure as a parent. Or a teenager may lie to her parents about her social activities because of a mistaken assumption that they wish to dictate every aspect of her life.

No logical, scientific basis can be established for such concepts as "family reality" or "family pathology," despite what many ecological or family therapists believe. Psychological problems, like medical disorders, can only arise within an individual human being. In some families each individual member may suffer from psychological problems; in other families only one member may have problems, even though the other members are influenced by that member. Some family therapists forget that the family is nothing more than the sum total of its members.

If the forms of therapy so far discussed rest upon irrational ideas, the *Dr. Shamans* of the world take these ideas to their ultimate conclusions. Such therapists claim to provide past-life regressions and other so-called out-of-body experiences for their clients. How? Nobody knows how, because such methods are based, at best, on vague and mystical delusions and, at worst, on fraud and deception. Dr. Shaman does not ask his clients to place trust in scientific principles or evidence; instead, he asks them to simply have faith. While this may not seem unusual for a religion or a cult, it is revolutionary for such activity to be categorized as science or medicine.

These approaches seem to gain a certain degree of professional credibility, especially as failures in other therapies lead to growing disappointment and desperation. Therapists such as Dr. Shaman often refer to their methods as focusing on "spiritual issues," meaning that their approach is based upon pure faith rather than evidence and proof. Of course, not all "spiritual" therapists go to the lengths of Dr. Shaman, but he does illustrate the undiluted version of any psychotherapy which does not anchor itself in rational scientific principles.

Last but not least, *Dr. Gloom-and-Doom* represents a relatively new breed of therapists who emphasize what they call the "inner child" and its influence on all adults. The "inner child" seems to refer to a series of inaccurate or distorted conclusions about oneself that an individual carries, subconsciously, to adulthood. The "inner child" approach to therapy must be given some credit for its valid points. Any therapist knows that childhood experiences can have a profound effect on the adult's later life.

The problem with the "inner child" approach is that it is victim-oriented. Conscientious graduates of "inner child" therapy tend to have a self-pitying approach to life. "My parents were mean to me, perhaps even abused me. So what do I do now?" seems to summarize their unspoken predicament. Inner child therapy, while making some valid points about the influence of certain parental behaviors (such as shaming or moralizing) on the young child, does not provide the victimized individual with a perspective about how to rise above such abuses. Vulnerable therapy clients need help in recognizing that no parent, however abusive or insensitive, can take away the adult's free will to think and act independently and, as a consequence, ultimately feel and behave differently.

Although I have discussed the most frequently practiced forms of therapy, I am not offering a comprehensive list of all psychotherapies. My attempt to summarize significant methods of psychotherapy, however, has left out another very important approach which is only beginning to show its influence on the therapy field: the *cognitive*.[5] Cognitive therapy is based on the idea that distorted, unrealistic thoughts lead to unhealthy negative emotions like depression and anxiety. When you learn to think about your problems in a more positive and realistic way, you can change the way you feel.[6] In order to understand and benefit from cognitive therapy, however, a client must adopt a rational philosophy of life, the focus of discussion in Chapter Three.

What Should I Expect of Psychotherapy?

Because numerous schools of psychotherapy exist, and most therapists use a mixture of approaches, it can be difficult for a prospective client to assess which methods a therapist is using. A better formula for evaluating psychotherapy from the consumer point-of-view is required. After over a decade of experience, discussion, and reflection on the subject, I have reached the conclusion that seven factors are essential to good therapy. Without the presence of all seven factors, the effectiveness of the therapy is seriously diminished.

I have developed these factors from clinical observation and logical reasoning. I have put them to the test in practice over and over again during hundreds of hours of therapy sessions with hundreds of different clients. I have also factored in the experiences of clients with other therapists, as well as the experiences of and discussions with therapists with whom I agree and disagree. I have considered the essential components of all forms of psychotherapy and evaluated them above and beyond the labels conventionally applied to them. These factors ought to prove helpful in evaluating one's current or potential therapist.

Factor One: *Feedback—not silence.* A therapist should talk to the client and have a dialogue with him. This point sounds like common sense, but many therapists appear to be highly passive and do not respond to their clients other than to nod "um-hmm" or occasionally to ask, "What do you think?" Horror stories of therapists falling asleep on their clients are not unheard of. Recently, attention has been focused on computer therapy, in which a computer program acts as the therapist. Even the most primitive computer could do a better job than therapists who fail to engage in a dialogue with their clients!

In daily practice, I encounter a surprising number of new clients who are seeking a different therapist because their last one did not speak to them, or did not offer them any specific feedback or guidelines. Bad experiences with silence generally indicate that clients were previously treated by a therapist using some version of the Freudian or neo-Freudian psychodynamic model. Such therapists are usually quiet because: (a) they see passivity as a therapeutic virtue to enhance the "transference" process; (b) through poor training they do not know what they are doing; or (c) they are emotionally drained and exhausted by their work. The point, however, remains—that therapists ought to engage in an active dialogue with their clients, even as they maintain professional detachment.

Factor Two: *Empowerment.* Empowerment consists of giving clients the psychological tools to take charge of their own lives, as quickly as possible. Empowerment means avoiding the false alternative of silence versus advice-giving. The classic Freudian therapist says little to his client. On the other hand, *Dear Abby,* and others like her, dispense advice with reckless simplicity. Good therapy does not fall into either of these traps. The good therapist operates on the premise that *human reason* is the best method for solving emotional problems, and that good therapists help their clients better use this capacity.

The advice giver, though usually well-intentioned, seeks to do the reasoning for the client. The silent therapist, on the other hand, encourages the client to *feel* his feelings but not to apply reason and thought to them. The good therapist neither reasons for his client nor ignores the fact that reason exists.

What exactly is reason? Human reason refers to the process of identifying facts of reality using one's capacity for sensation and perception (sight, smell, taste, hearing, and touch) and abstract conceptualization. Conceptualization involves the condensation of many bits and pieces of perceptions into more generalized, theoretical knowledge. Reason is the method by which a human being integrates the data perceived by his senses into abstract concepts.

We share our sensation and perception abilities with other animals, like dogs and cats, but the ability to form abstract concepts, such as "honesty," "career" or "country" is uniquely human. Conceptualization, however elementary or complex, represents a capacity open to virtually all human beings, from a young child to Albert Einstein. When a child grasps that all flat surfaces with four legs are tables, he has formed the concept "table." When a young adult grasps that there exist standards of right and wrong and each implies certain consequences, she forms the concept "justice." When Einstein grasped the concept of relativity, he engaged in a highly advanced level of concept formation.[7]

Good therapy is an empowerment process. Good therapists empower their clients by encouraging them to rely on independent, logical judgment. They are neither remote and passive nor authoritarian and controlling. A good therapist wants to help the client better understand the relationship between thoughts and emotions and, as a consequence, to discover the origins of one's psychological problems.

Factor Three: *Focus on reality—not simply one's feelings.* A good therapist assumes, and encourages the client to assume, that feelings are not necessarily facts. Feelings are an automatic response to an object, event or person one perceives. Feelings are not bad; nor are they, by themselves, a means of discovering the truth about any issue.

If one is depressed, for example, one needs to identify the thoughts and conclusions which have led to the feeling that life is hopeless and worthless. This process may be difficult, and, for a depressed individual, usually requires the help of a good therapist. A good therapist has the following attitude: "I'm sincerely sorry you feel life is awful. Can you prove to me that life *is* awful? Let's first discover what the facts really are, and whether or not the feelings you have correspond to the facts." If the client's life turns out to be, in fact, awful, then the therapist helps the client discover reasonable solutions for improving it.

A bad therapist mistakenly sees feelings, by themselves, as a means of defining reality and proving a point: "If you feel that your husband is victimizing you, then he is. After all, aren't all men brutes? If you feel that your parents are abusing you, they must be. After all, aren't all children victims of their parents' emotional abuse?"

Clients in therapy must keep in mind that the process of thought and reason, with the therapist's help, provides the validation (or invalidation) of feelings. Feelings may arise from a whole series of assumptions and conclusions, some of which may be correct and others of which may be mistaken. Granted, human logic is not infallible. At the same time, substituting feelings for careful, logical deliberation is no more productive in one's private, emotional life than in the professional or scientific world.

Factor Four: *Solution-focused therapy.* All therapy, whether it lasts for one session, one year or five years needs to be solution-focused. Solution-focused therapy emphasizes the client's unique strengths and ability to solve problems using his own judgment.

In solution-focused therapy, treatment contracts are common. Some understanding about outcome—whether written or verbal, broad or specific—must exist between therapist and client, and needs to be reevaluated at selected intervals. Therapy can go seriously adrift if therapist and client do not have a clear, mutual understanding of the expected outcome. Both therapist and client need to understand and agree upon the expected results of therapy.

Completion of the following statement helps a therapy client determine expected outcome: *At the end of therapy, I will.* . . . Consider several examples. "At the end of therapy, I will make a decision about which job I want to take." "At the end of therapy, my husband and I will have a better idea of how to fight fairly and rationally." "At the end of therapy, I will have improved self-esteem, which means that I will question my decisions less, stop second-guessing myself so much, and not jump to the conclusion that others are criticizing me when, in fact, they may not be." "At the end of therapy, I will feel less depressed and approach life with a more positive, realistic attitude."

In agreeing upon expected outcome, I advise psychotherapy clients to beware of vague or open-ended contracts, especially ones worded exclusively by the therapist. Common examples include: to "get through" a life transition; to "deal with" certain problems; to "work through" issues of co-dependency, shaming, abandonment, early childhood experiences, and so on. If I were a psychotherapy client unfamiliar with such terms and I were paying good money to the therapist who uses them, I would want to know the meaning of "abandonment," "deal with," and "working through."

If a therapist uses vague or nonspecific terms, and the client has no idea what they mean, the therapeutic alliance is seriously affected. If a client does ask, and the therapist responds with evasiveness or defensiveness, then a healthy therapeutic alliance may be impossible.

Good therapists want to answer their clients' questions.

Factor Five: *A Systems Perspective.* A good therapist recognizes that all therapy has some kind of impact on those around the client. He recognizes that all individuals live in an external context which influences, but does not have to determine, his ideas, emotions and behaviors.

The "system" refers to the client's household, family, friends, co-workers, and larger social, economic, and cultural institutions which affect his daily life. A systemic therapist recognizes the importance of external influences on the client's life, especially of family members who may be complicating the client's problems. For example, a teenage girl's runaway behavior may be due to the alcoholism of a father who beats and molests her. "Family" therapists and "systems" therapists refer to essentially the same type of mental health professional.

A systems therapist maintains a perspective about the environment or context in which a client lives. If a woman complains that her husband does not pay enough attention to her, a good therapist realizes that the husband also has a point of view and his point of view must be considered. A good therapist understands that a recent immigrant from a family- and duty-oriented culture may have different assumptions about raising teenagers from a parent who wants her child to eventually leave the family and develop his own career and make his own choices. A good therapist is able to see that, as one individual in a family or relationship improves, another family member may (at least temporarily) feel threatened, and efforts are made to identify this fact if it occurs. A systems perspective means that the therapist anticipates the reaction of family members to the client's therapy, and even considers inviting them to sessions with the client's consent.

It may seem that I am contradicting my earlier criticism of the ecological therapist, who often calls himself a family or systemic therapist. Unfortunately labels, often improperly applied because of confusion and misunderstanding, can distract one from the essential point. A critical distinction must be made between an ecological therapist and a good, systemic therapist. The legitimate systemic therapist recognizes that, while environmental factors are important, they do not *determine* the outcome of an individual life. A victim of sexual abuse, for example, can learn to recognize that the abuse was wrong and led her to develop self-destructive attitudes regarding sexuality. She can choose to identify and change these self-destructive thoughts and feelings within a reasonable period of time. She need not become a permanent victim.

To avoid the confusion over therapeutic labels, it is better to judge a therapist by his actions than by the labels he attaches to himself.

Factor Six: *Alliance—not advocacy.* A good therapist should want the client to improve his life and be fully committed to helping him to do so. Such an alliance serves both the client's and the therapist's interest.

However, this sense of being on the client's side should not compromise either the objectivity or the detachment of a therapist. A therapist is neither one's lawyer nor one's friend. The client's relationship with his therapist should, generally speaking, be confined to the office or the telephone. Although the therapeutic alliance is not the mystical relationship encouraged by the Freudians, it is nevertheless unwise to extend it outside of the therapeutic context. The alliance, while superficially resembling a friendship, remains one-sided because the therapist does not discuss her own problems or concerns with the client.

Therapeutic advocacy refers to a wider concept in which the therapist holds "siding" with the client as a primary value, even to the point of patronizing the client. Advocacy, of course, may express itself in psychological as well as legal form.

A good therapist seeks to be honest—in a nice, respectful, clinical way, but honest nevertheless. A client does not have to agree with the therapist. At the same time, a good therapist explains how he reached his conclusions. If a client's therapist believes that the client may be trying to take the easy way out by sending her teenage son to a boarding school, for example, he owes it to the client to tell her this and explain why.

In my experience, certain individuals are attracted to jobs in the psychotherapy field because of chips they have carried on their shoulders for decades. Perhaps they are angry about perceived injustices from their own childhoods and channel this anger into their work. A therapist who was sexually molested as a child may believe that everyone is a victim of some sort, and sees the rest of the world as potential aggressors, even when there is no logic or evidence to support such a view.

The danger of such therapists does not lie in the fact that they were victimized as children. Such victimizations do not prevent an individual from becoming a competent and objective therapist. The danger lies in the lack of objectivity and reason with which chronically angry therapists approach clients whose lives resemble their own.

If overzealous advocacy is inappropriate, then what is the alternative? A recognition of the idea of therapeutic alliance. The relationship between therapist and client is not primarily one of support. The primary job of the therapist is to help the client examine his life situation or emotional experiences more rationally and objectively. Good therapists want to help clients understand things as they are, not necessarily as the client feels them to be. Someone once said to me, "People pay therapists *not* to care." This is true. A client should expect the therapist to comment on or question statements, emotions, and behaviors in a respectful and competent but also an honest manner. This is the meaning of therapy viewed as an alliance rather than as advocacy.

Factor Seven: *Integration of past and present.* Bad therapy rests on the premise that an individual's childhood experiences shaped him in ways that are largely beyond his control in adult life. Good therapy rests on the premise that one's childhood experiences, no matter how traumatic, are entirely reversible through conscious choice and effort.

The following statement illustrates the thoughts of a person influenced by a deterministic, victim-oriented therapist: "My mother preached to me. My father beat me. My brother made fun of me. I am the adult child of a dysfunctional family. I have special needs. I must let people know of my dysfunction and insist that they meet my special needs. In a way, I am disabled. I must accept this disability and learn to live the best life I possibly can. Above all, I must hold myself in unconditional positive regard in order to develop and maintain self-esteem. I must also demand unconditional acceptance from others at all times. Nobody has a right to judge me."

The thoughts of a person influenced by good therapy might be summed up this way: "My mother preached to me. My father beat me. My brother made fun of me. My introduction to life was not a pretty one. It led me to think that life *has* to be a constant series of conflicts and that most individuals will not respect me and treat me well. Now that I am an adult, however, I recognize that these conclusions were erroneous. Life need not be full of obstacles and pain, as it was in childhood. If a boyfriend abuses me, I have the freedom to send him on his way. He is not my father. Furthermore, I know that there are plenty of people in the world who are not abusive, and I will search them out and keep them in my life. I will never settle for abusive individuals in my personal life. I am not duty-bound to live my life for others as a martyr. On the other hand, I *am* responsible for developing my potential, because only through the development of my strengths and abilities can I hope to achieve happiness. I must earn and constantly work for happiness, and I need not fear the evaluations or criticisms of others so long as I rely on my own judgment in everything I do."

The first approach states that there is little an individual can do about her early experiences—other than to identify them and insist that others in her life realize they have disabled and victimized her. The second approach suggests that while she does *not* have control over early childhood experiences, she does have control over the way she thinks and acts in the present. Although there may be errors or distortions in her thinking and the right conclusions are not always immediately apparent to her, once she identifies such distortions she can modify her emotional responses over time.

If someone is currently in psychotherapy, especially if he has been in treatment for a number of months or years,

I advise him to ask himself which premise best summarizes the basis for his therapy. If the first, then the individual's therapist has failed to teach him to integrate the past and the present. While such therapy may help him gain more insight about his past, it will not do much to help him in the present. In good therapy, the past is viewed as a means of providing information to help the client live with more contentment in the present.

A Few Words of Caution

I want to stress two points.

First of all, the term "bad therapist" does not necessarily imply a moral judgment. I take it for granted that most therapists mean well and that dishonest or abusive therapists will, over the long run, expose themselves through their work.

"Bad therapist" refers to an individual who practices psychotherapy derived from mistaken principles. Whether the therapist knows the therapy is bad is another story. If a client is able to conclude, beyond a reasonable doubt, that his therapist practices inappropriate methods, then he should not continue with the therapist, even if he sees the therapist as a decent person.

Good intentions cannot counteract bad methods. Should an incompetent car mechanic fix the brakes on one's car? Bad therapy can do more harm than no therapy. Bad therapy often feeds into today's social problems, rather than reducing them, because it reinforces the false view that logic and feelings cannot be brought into successful harmony with one another.

Underlying the practice of bad therapy is the philosophical view of determinism. To restate, the philosophy of determinism argues that we are all helpless victims shaped exclusively by external causes whether it be our childhood, our racial, gender, or socioeconomic status, or other factors. Under the influence of determinism, too many clients arrive at the therapist's office with the impression that they need to passively sit back and have something done to them, instead of being held responsible for actively thinking about their feelings and learning how to develop reasonable solutions to their problems.

Of course individuals are influenced by external factors. At the same time, *individual choice* must never be left out of any assessment of human nature, especially psychology. Without recognition of choice, we will develop into a culture of unthinking, passive agents devoid of innovation, creativity, and individuality.

Bad Therapy—
And How It Can Hurt
the Client

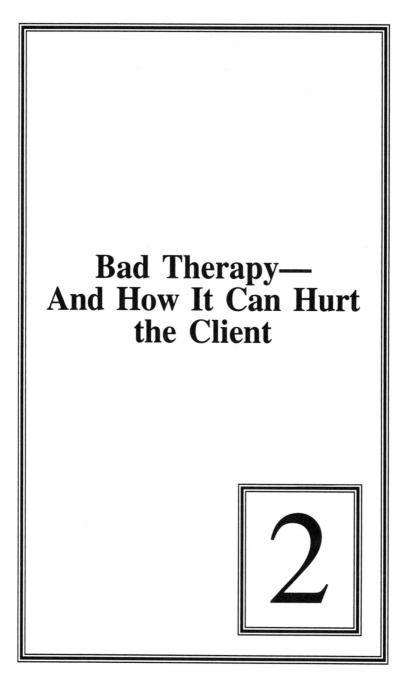

2

Is any kind of help better than nothing? So long as a therapist means well, should a client feel safe? Is good or bad therapy simply a matter of opinion?

No.

In psychotherapy, a Pandora's box of emotions, unresolved pain, and long-forgotten issues typically invade a client's consciousness. If therapy is to be effective, it will lead a person to think, feel, and behave differently. Simply talking about one's problems, with no sense of direction or conscious purpose, does not guarantee mental health. What the therapist says and how she presents it are important factors. The theoretical orientation upon which the therapy rests determines how both therapist and client approach it.

Good therapy relies on the premise of psychological individualism: the idea that no better means exists for evaluating oneself or the external world than a calm and deliberate process of thought.

Feelings are not enough, by themselves, to identify the facts of existence. The *feeling* that the world is a hopeless place or that nothing good will ever happen does not make it so. Feelings need to be subjected to logical reasoning before they can be adequately verified or rejected.

Human beings need to take responsibility for asking themselves questions about their feelings. If they do not, they gradually become overwhelmed and, usually without realizing it, begin to assume that their anxious or depressed feelings represent facts. Simple "self-talk" techniques can help the individual deal with such feelings as these: "I feel that I am worthless. Is this really the case? Can I provide evidence which warrants this emotional conclusion? If so, then I need to figure out some strategies for resolving this problem. At the same time, I cannot accept it as a fact, unless I first see persuasive and conclusive evidence."

Aside from encouraging rational thought, good therapy also rests on the idea that self-reliance is a virtue. Psychotherapy is a means to an end. The end includes greater self-reliance, individualism, self-esteem, and rejection of the idea that one owes any aspect of one's life or self to others. "How can you act or think differently, so that you can better go it alone?" is the basic message good therapists impart to their clients. Good therapists want their clients to improve as quickly as possible.

To better illustrate the importance of self-reliance and rational thought, I will first provide some common examples of ineffective therapy based upon opposite concepts. In chapter one, I described seven essential characteristics of good therapy. In the sections which follow, I will elaborate on each of these characteristics and explain why their absence can lead to harmful long-term effects.

The Consequences of Silence

Silent therapists provide nothing except an occasional nod or the question, "How does that make you feel?" If they have any opinions or reactions to what the client says, the client rarely hears about them. The client may find the silence irritating. She might wonder if the therapist really listens or cares about what she says.

Silent therapy can have many consequences. First and foremost is the effect on the client's self-esteem. Many individuals seek help because they feel worthless. They experience frustration with life and they want to know what, if anything, they can do about it.

Given this scenario, what happens if they seek help from a therapist who never gives them any feedback? Individuals with some self-esteem will be properly disgusted by this waste of time and money, and terminate the process before it gets out of hand. Individuals with little self-esteem may conclude that, since the therapist has credentials and is experienced, he must know something most of the world does not know. Clients often see therapists as wiser and more knowledgeable than any one human can possibly be. They sometimes feel, incorrectly, that therapists are capable of judging their worth or capability better than anyone else, including themselves. In the eyes of the vulnerable therapy client, the silent therapist exudes an aura of power and omniscience.

A second consequence of silent therapy involves disappointed expectations. Most individuals initially approach psychotherapy with a heightened, even exaggerated, sense of hope. While the client's expectations of the therapist need to conform to reality, the person who earnestly seeks help ought to expect to get it. After all, you expect that an accountant will help you solve your tax dilemma, and you expect that your doctor will help you treat your sore throat. When confronted with the silent therapist, the conscientious therapy client may become disappointed and not seek help again. He may jump to the conclusion that because one therapist seems incompetent, no one can help him. The practice of silent psychotherapy leads many of its victims to conclude, inaccurately, that all mental health treatment is a sham.

Silent therapy, for those who choose to endure it, also leads to an overall sense of uncertainty. For example, the client might experience relief from discussing his thoughts and feelings, but receives no feedback from the therapist regarding appropriate strategies for solving a particular problem. If the therapist never defines his treatment philosophy, then it becomes difficult to assess when and how to end therapy.

A therapist who does not ask the client, "How will we know therapy is over?" may not know or care to answer this question. The client can therefore assume that no therapeutic purpose exists, except to give the client someone with whom to talk. At the most, silent therapists may encourage clients to vaguely "work through" some issues that might, in some indirect, unspecified, or accidental way lead to an improved state of mental health. "Working through" issues is a common psychotherapeutic expression, but it often is not clear to the client (or perhaps the therapist) what this vague process actually involves.

Aside from a sense of uncertainty, another consequence of silent therapy is the high probability that it will not lead to a reduction in symptoms. Psychotherapy requires a sense of purpose as much as other human endeavors. Consider a road map analogy as an illustration. Suppose that you live in New York and decide to drive to California without the use of either a road map or road signs. You may get there eventually, but not as the result of any conscious or logical process. The same concept applies to silent, unfocused therapy. In silent therapy, no objective for determining a successful outcome (from either the therapist's or the client's perspective) exists. The therapist provides no hint that one is necessary.

Clients in silent therapy should not let this issue go undiscussed. First, they should identify their expectations of therapy and then address the issue with the therapist directly. The resulting reaction will reveal much about the therapist's ethical standards and professional competence.

If the therapist reacts in an evasive or hostile manner, the client should be concerned. If the therapist does not react with evasiveness or hostility, but remains unable to help the client chart a more conscious course for therapy, then no successful outcome should be anticipated.

Whether or not the therapist is a good or kind human being is beside the point. No matter how well-intentioned a therapist, he cannot save the client from a bad therapeutic method. Many therapists are wrapped up in bad therapeutic methods and philosophies and do not know, any more than their clients, how to untangle themselves. Terminating with an ineffective therapist is better than risking continued exposure to an approach based on principles which ignore the important human need to set goals, to focus, and to learn how to separate distortive emotions from logical facts.

The Consequences of Advice-Oriented Therapy

Opinionated, bossy therapists often mean well, but they have an irritating habit of interrupting and telling a person what she should know instead of letting her figure out solutions for herself. In extreme cases, one may even wonder if such therapists are more interested in hearing themselves talk than in empowering their clients. Who needs to hire a professional for giving advice, when the client can most probably find such individuals in her personal life free of charge?

Advice-oriented therapy rests on the implicit, and usually unintended, assumption that the client is incapable of discovering answers or insights on her own. The therapist seeks to pound ideas into the client's head rather than allow her to consider, evaluate and, only if truly convinced, eventually internalize them as her own.

Contrary to popular impressions, good therapists do not give their clients advice. Good therapists help their clients learn how to form their own opinions and then act on them. Good therapists communicate the following message implicitly, through their actions and statements: "Maybe you should do such-and-such *because....*"

Advice-giving therapists, however, operate under a very different implicit framework: "Do such-and-such because I say so. Trust me. It's good for you." Whether benign or dictatorial, advice-oriented therapy is authoritarian in nature because it relies upon commands, rather than carefully and logically reasoned conclusions, as a therapeutic method. Since human thought processes cannot be forced, and conclusions can only be accepted by a client if she clearly understands and agrees with them, authoritarian approaches do not work.

As an illustration of this point, consider the young child first learning mathematics in grade school. Does the teacher work all of the problems for the child? Or does she do selected problems in the beginning to help the child learn the underlying principles of addition and subtraction, and then allow the child to try some on his own? Psychotherapy follows the same idea. The therapist does, on occasion, provide answers and feedback, but always with explanations attached. Until the client grasps the therapist's reasoning for making a certain point, the client remains unable to apply the point.

Another potentially harmful consequence of advice-oriented therapy is that the client will develop an unhealthy dependence on both the therapy and the therapist. The client will think that therapy is working, unaware of the most important task of any therapy: helping him gain more confidence in his own reasoning abilities and his independent judgment, so that he eventually will no longer need professional help.

Advice-oriented therapy teaches the client how to memorize solutions without understanding them. Like the student whose teacher does all his math problems for him, the client is set free into the world with only a vague sense of how to cope. When confronted with an issue, instead of asking himself, "How do I apply the method my therapist taught me to this situation?" the question becomes: "What would my therapist tell me to do in this situation?"

Advice-oriented therapy, if identified in time, need not result in failure. The client might consider telling his therapist that, while he really appreciates the advice, he also wants to learn how to generate such solutions on his own. Perhaps the therapist might teach him the basic principles which underlie the advice. A principle is a general rule which can be applied to many specific situations. An example of a principle is the idea that feelings are not necessarily facts, and that one needs to rationally examine one's feelings before acting on them.

If the therapist reacts favorably to such a request and commits to working with the client on learning more general principles about staying mentally healthy, then the client can satisfactorily continue with the same therapist. If the therapist refuses or is unable to change, then the client ought to pursue other avenues.

The Consequences of Feeling-Centered Therapy

Feeling-centered therapy encourages clients to identify and act exclusively on feelings. This form of therapy creates or reinforces the false assumption that feelings are on an equal par with, if not superior to, reason and logic as a method for knowing what is going on in the world.

There is no substitute for logic as a method of coping with unexplained or troubling emotions. Logic is a method of identifying facts and resolving contradictions. Logic is an intimidating word to most people. Logical people are often thought to be cold, callous, and indifferent to other human beings. Nevertheless, to be logical does not mean to ignore or repress one's feelings; being logical means checking to see if one's feelings correspond to the facts.

Despite the existence of logic, most psychotherapies still rest on the stipulation that feelings represent a viable method of assessing, judging, or evaluating a situation. The mistaken ideas underlying bad therapy increasingly expand beyond the therapist's office. Sometimes therapists, especially the sort who appear on highly influential day-time talk shows, go so far as to claim that one's feelings, and feelings alone, embody the essence of being "human." College students, under the influence of psychology and other humanities professors, increasingly place a higher value on unexamined emotions at the expense of logic, facts and reason. As John Leo of *U.S. News & World Report* has written, "The radical subjectivity sweeping through education has many sources, but the most easily understood version of it comes from therapy: Feelings take precedence over facts and norms. 'If you feel that the whole world is on top of you, then it is,' in the words of one college student. And if you feel that you are a victim of hate speech or harassment, the feeling itself is conclusive evidence that you are right. In the world of feelings, the indictment is the conviction. But what happens to society when everyone is encouraged to think like this?"[8]

If the feeling-centered view were true, then all depressed people ought to kill themselves at once. After all, if they *feel* that life is worthless, then the feeling must be true. The notion that feelings constitute an adequate definition of reality seems absurd to any sane person. Nevertheless, a growing number of therapists perpetuate this very notion.

I have encountered adults who feel that they were abused as children simply because their parents hurt their feelings, conclusions they drew from daily contact with popular television talk shows. I encounter an increasing number of parents terrified of hurting their child's feelings, even if the child needs to be corrected. These parents have the impression, from our therapy-soaked and feeling-dominated culture, that hurt feelings in childhood lead to low self-esteem and failure in adulthood. I spend countless therapy hours trying to undo the damage of such ideas.

Sometimes feelings correspond to reality (e.g., depression over the death of a child) and sometimes they do not (e.g., terror that there is a monster under one's bed). Regardless of feelings, facts continue to exist and impose their consequences on all who fail to accept their relevance.

Feelings can become harmful if used to make decisions without any reference to logic, reason, and proof. Consequently, therapies which emphasize "feel, feel" at the expense of "what do I *do* with these feelings once I know them?" do not help clients solve problems.

A therapist who encourages the client to look inward and introspect, especially if the client habitually ignores his feelings, performs a valuable service. The therapist who never teaches the client how to think and reason about feelings inflicts harm on those he intends to help. The client's powerful emotions of anger, sadness, or hurt have been reactivated; but, without rational techniques, the client has no idea what to do with them.

Although feelings can be mistaken, to acknowledge them in a therapist's office is much healthier than continuing to ignore them. At the same time, a client should not be misled into thinking that feelings are equivalent to facts. Most feeling-centered therapists seem unwilling or unable to recognize this latter point. The increases in divorce, family instability, and racial/sexual tensions may be aggravated by the influence of feeling-centered therapists who fail to teach clients how to reason with their emotions. Perhaps if more therapists taught their clients methods for thinking prior to acting, instead of merely ruminating on emotions, social problems would improve.

Feelings, because they happen automatically and with lightning-like speed, often will amplify or exaggerate the facts. If Sue's husband forgets to take out the garbage for the second night in row, her emotions might lead her to the overgeneralization that her husband does not care about her. But once she calms down, she can consider the full context of the situation and recognize that, despite her husband's lapse, he still cares. The ability to see the difference between one's immediate reaction and one's logically reasoned conclusion is often referred to as a sense of perspective. Good therapy encourages the development of a rational perspective.

Feeling-centered therapy fails to encourage individuals to develop or maintain a sense of perspective. In some cases, I have seen individuals who previously had a sense of perspective lose it altogether because of the influences of their feeling-centered therapist. I am willing to give most feeling-centered therapists the benefit of the doubt and assume that they genuinely believe they are helping their clients. At the same time, prospective clients need to recognize that well-intentioned, feeling-centered therapy can become a harmful experience.

If a client comes to accept the feeling-centered premise, then he will attempt to make decisions based on gut feelings without reference to facts known to exist independent of subjective experience. He might, for instance, decide to quit his job on a feeling that he no longer likes it, without weighing the consequences of the decision. In another case, he might decide to embark on an extramarital love affair on a feeling that it is right for him without carefully considering the long-term impact of such a relationship. The good therapist helps him focus on the long-term consequences of his actions, not simply on the strong feelings racing through his consciousness at any given moment.

Of course, no therapist labels him- or herself "feeling-centered." Feeling-centered therapists often mean well and have no conception of how destructive their methods are. Clients in feeling-centered therapy can ask their therapist to give them more guidance on what to do with their feelings once they have identified them by asking, "Should I only act on my feelings? If not, then what criteria can I use to know when to act on them and when not to do so? Are feelings the only way of knowing the truth? If not, then how can I learn to distinguish feelings from reality?" The therapist's responses to such questions, as well as the degree of hostility or evasion he displays when confronted with them, will help in assessing both the therapist's methodology and professional integrity.

Consequences of Unfocused Therapy

Unfocused therapy fails to finish the sentence: "At the end of treatment I will. . . . " The medical analogy to unfocused therapy involves a client's going to a doctor once a week for no particular reason. The client solicits help in "working through" any physiological issues which might "come up" for him; or, perhaps he learns to understand his childhood diseases (or, better still, the childhood diseases of his parents and grandparents). While certain essential differences between the processes of psychotherapy and medical treatment obviously exist, this fact by no means justifies the rationalization that mental health treatment need not have specific, definable goals.

Preposterous as it might seem, much of today's psychotherapy still operates under the framework that talking is always an end in itself. The negative consequences of such an approach do not always appear obvious to the therapy client. Without an expected outcome of treatment, how can progress be assessed? How can there be progress if there is no goal? While the neurotic characters played by Woody Allen in the movies may find nothing wrong with open-ended approaches to therapy, conscientious individuals in search of genuine emotional resolution have reason to feel disappointed and even betrayed.

I often receive referrals for clients with previous treatment failures. While I always give prior therapists the benefit of the doubt, I must admit to being appalled by some of the following complaints: "How am I supposed to solve my job problems by talking about my parents' marriage for months on end?" "What do my grade school experiences have to do with what's going on in my life right now?" "I spent a year with a psychotherapist, meeting twice a week, and I still have no idea what therapy is supposed to do for me."

Individuals with such complaints are most likely the victims of unfocused therapy. Unfocused therapy has no beginning, middle or end. It simply reacts to situations as they occur. There are no principles to guide it other than the unstated assumption that talking out one's problems will somehow eliminate them.

Why is unfocused therapy so commonplace? Many individuals who seek psychological help are motivated by a vague sense of wanting to feel better without being sure how to know when they are better. For such individuals, bad therapy quickly becomes part of the problem rather than part of the solution. The failure of such clients to focus on long-range goals throughout all areas of their lives probably caused a major share of their unhappiness in the first place. A good therapist will spot this pattern immediately and ask the client to develop a short-term, easily solved goal before moving on to harder ones.

A bad therapist will not address the problem at all. Instead, he will simply drift along with the client in hopes that a better tomorrow will eventually arrive. If it does, therapy is seen as a success. If the better tomorrow never arrives and the client becomes frustrated, he is wryly dismissed as "not ready" for psychotherapy.

An individual with unrealistic expectations of himself (an unreasonable perfectionist, for example) is particularly vulnerable to unfocused therapy. A good therapist will spot such unrealistic self-assessments early on and encourage the client to examine them prior to solving any other problems. This self-examination helps the client develop realistic expectations so therapy has a chance of succeeding. In bad therapy, unfortunately, the client's basic problem will not be spotted, and he will likely blame future treatment disappointments on his own alleged inadequacies.

Perhaps the worst consequence of unfocused therapy is that it allows the therapist, instead of the client, to set the agenda for session discussions. Consider a patient who goes to a doctor for a broken leg. Now imagine how he feels if the doctor does not seem concerned about his broken leg, but prefers to talk about the patient's arthritis instead. Imagine if the doctor only wanted to discuss the patient's family history of arthritis! This example exaggerates only slightly the futility of working with a therapist who relies on an unfocused approach.

I do not mean to imply that psychotherapy is equivalent to medical treatment. Treatment of medical problems usually requires extreme passivity on the part of the patient. Typically, the doctor provides the patient with a diagnosis and suggests a specific treatment. The patient need only sit back and follow recommendations about diet, rest, and so forth. Good psychotherapy, on the other hand, requires human will and initiative. In psychotherapy, the client must make the *choice* to change, while the therapist stands near by, coaching and offering feedback when necessary.

Psychotherapy entails much more of a team effort than traditional medical treatment. A medical patient can be coerced into surgery, for example, if he is restrained and knocked out in time. Nobody can be coerced into psychotherapy, beyond dragging him—kicking and screaming—into the therapist's office. The therapist must be willing to help; the client must be willing to *accept* help.

In addition to the issue of coercion, therapists disagree on whether therapy ought to treat the root causes or the symptoms of mental disorder. Traditionally, the root causes of mental disorder are thought to involve unresolved feelings from one's childhood. Symptoms, on the other hand, refer to current feelings of depression, anxiety, hostility, etc. To favor either side of this issue involves accepting a false alternative. To imply that one must choose between symptom reduction and root causes seems preposterous. Why can't good therapy strive for both?

In this respect, a highly motivated client and a good therapist can prove a powerful match. I have seen clients make dramatic insights into their childhood within five or ten sessions and then use this knowledge to better appreciate themselves as adults with choices and control over their lives. The simple recognition of "that was then, this is now" can often have more impact than hours and hours of therapy.

The Consequences of
Tunnel-Vision Therapy

Tunnel-vision therapy refers to any form of psychotherapy which fails to consider the larger context of the individual client's life. The larger context includes relevant influences such as spouse, children, parents, close friends, and family members who are part of the individual's personal social system. While such individuals need not always be included in the treatment itself, most therapists tend to underestimate the value of doing so.

Good *or* bad therapy almost always has an affect on those close to the client, especially over time. Most therapists recognize this fact, but few will share this knowledge or help the client prepare to deal with it. As an actual or prospective therapy client, one ought to be aware that the option of inviting a family member, spouse, or other relevant person exists.

Occasionally, individuals will invite "significant others" to their sessions if the focus of therapy consists of a conflict between the two parties. Sometimes it is not advisable to invite outside parties to therapy. Either way, individuals close to the client are often affected by the therapy, especially if the treatment is effective and leads to changes in the client's personality or behaviors. I label the reactions of "significant others" as therapeutic side effects.

Therapeutic side effects need not be harmful. In fact, side effects tend to do harm only when clients fail to identify them as a normal part of psychotherapeutic treatment. A husband, for instance, might sincerely want his wife to overcome her fear of driving. However, if she becomes more independent as a result of therapy, he may feel threatened and lash out at her in some way. The wife in turn may rush to the conclusion that he seeks to control her. In reality, the husband may simply be scared of losing her. While therapeutic side-effects are not always quite so dramatic, they are nearly always present. Good therapists work very hard to prepare clients for them ahead of time and respond in a respectful, realistic way if the need arises.

Tunnel-vision therapists ignore or downplay therapeutic side-effects. If a therapist does not take into account the effect that therapy can have on persons close to the client, he does the client a disservice. If a man discusses his wife's hostile attitude toward his therapy, for example, and the therapist ignores or downplays those reactions, then the therapist places added strains on the marriage. A therapist who deliberately ignores or belittles such factors fails to appreciate the larger context in which the client lives and shows ignorance of the powerful effect that therapy can have on the unintended "clients," particularly spouses.

Consider the case of the therapist who recommended to her female client that she take better care of herself. She suggested that the woman join a health club and take more time to rest at the end of the day. The client did so, but noticed over time that her husband resented such activities. She told her therapist that her husband was being unfair and making snide remarks about her new activities and about the therapist.

A good therapist would give the husband the benefit of the doubt. Perhaps the client was misreading her husband's motives, or misinterpreting his feelings, the therapist might suggest. Maybe the husband really was jealous, and he wished he could learn how to better take care of himself as well. Perhaps he was worried that as his wife became healthier and more attractive she would leave him for another man. Maybe, in fact, he was emotionally abusive and wanted to keep his wife under his control.

No competent therapist would encourage her client to arrive at this last conclusion without first ruling out all other explanations and inviting the husband in for one or several sessions. It can help both the client and the spouse to address this issue as a normal reaction to change, before leaping to conclusions about the moral character of the husband or the quality of the marriage.

The bad therapist's error, in such a case, would consist of taking everything the wife said at face value. An anti-male therapist, for example, operating on the false prejudice that all men are to some extent childish and irrational (see chapter five), would tend to agree with the client without making any attempt to discover the husband's point of view. While his actions may not necessarily be reasonable, perhaps they arose from insecurity and mistaken assumptions such as, "My wife will leave me if she starts to feel better about herself." Such a therapist might encourage her client to take a belligerent stance with her husband, or reinforce her client's feelings against her husband without encouraging her to evaluate them objectively. In the process, there could be damage done to the marriage and an otherwise preventable break-up might occur.

A tunnel-vision approach to psychotherapy can encourage the client to inappropriately see herself as fully responsible for her problem. If a client seeks therapy for emotional distress arising out of her husband's compulsive drinking, the therapist may see the client individually with no attempt to involve the husband. Consequently, the client might come to view the problem as entirely her fault. I am not criticizing therapists who treat spouses of alcoholics individually, since, under many circumstances, this may be preferable to dragging an unwilling spouse into therapy. On the other hand, good therapists might at least obtain confirmation that the spouse will participate in some form of treatment. At a minimum, the good therapist makes clear to the client that the husband's self-destructive choices are something for which he alone bears responsibility.

More often than unwilling spouses, reluctant and frightened children and teenagers are dragged to child psychologists, who treat the child with little or no effort to solicit the parents' and siblings' points of view. Such cases offer examples of tunnel-vision therapy at its worst. My experience has shown that many adults were forced into therapy as children and felt blamed for problems that, in hindsight, had more to do with the parents than with themselves. This observation should not imply, of course, that parents are always to "blame" for their child's behavior. Nevertheless, it remains virtually impossible to assess any child or teenager's problem outside the context of the family itself.

The Consequences of Advocacy-Oriented Therapy

Advocacy-oriented therapists, like advice-oriented therapists, want to act for the client, instead of letting the client act for himself. In advocacy-oriented therapy, the therapist extends this approach outside of the therapy office, either in a legal or a social context. Advocacy-oriented therapists testify for their clients in court. They tell a client's boss that the client cannot work, for an indefinite period, because of overwhelming emotions. They tell a client's husband that his wife cannot have sex for an indefinite period because of sexual abuse memories. They are often paternalistic and presumptuous, happily obliging the client's requests to take over or make important decisions for him.

Sometimes mental health professionals must interact with legal or social institutions. Although psychotherapists should not pose as legal experts, they cannot place themselves above the law either. Therapists are required, both legally and ethically, to report sexual or physical abuse of children when they have evidence that their client is guilty of such an offense. They also must warn potential victims of a client with homicidal intent. If a judge or court sees fit to subpoena a client's record, the therapist has to act in accord with laws regarding patient-doctor privilege.

Advocacy-oriented therapy does not, however, arise in a context of obeying the law and respecting ethical guidelines. Its context is more psychological than ethical or legal. Advocacy-oriented therapy involves a bond between client and therapist resting on two subconscious, unacknowledged assumptions: (1) you (the client) need me (the therapist); and (2) I (the therapist) need you (the client) to need me.

Of course, all psychotherapists "need" their clients if they wish to stay in business and continue to achieve personal and professional fulfillment. Both of these aims are legitimate. All clients need their therapists to help them with their problems. If clients did not need their therapists, they would not be participating in psychotherapy.

In advocacy-oriented therapy, however, the therapist holds the assumption that his self-worth relies upon others' dependence on him. This assumption represents a problem with which numerous psychotherapists are afflicted. Some refer to such a problem as a "rescuing" complex. Many therapists come to realize the dysfunctional nature of the rescuing complex. Others do not become fully aware of the issue, and as a result develop an unhealthy economic and psychological dependence on their clients.

Do all therapists who become legally involved with their clients, other than when required by law, suffer from a need to be needed? Not necessarily, but such involvement illustrates a clear warning signal.

A particularly dangerous therapist-client match exists between an advocacy-oriented therapist and a client who desperately needs to be liked. A reasonably healthy and competent therapist will spot the client's obsessive need to be liked early on in the therapy and help the client identify this mistaken assumption so that it may be recognized and changed. Unfortunately, the unhealthy therapist is unwilling and perhaps unable to help such a client identify an issue which he himself has not yet resolved. Instead, the therapist will communicate, through his excessive desire to help the client, that the client must be psychologically dependent on him in order to win and maintain the therapist's approval. The client senses this implicit psychological deal and, having a need to please everybody, including the therapist, will happily comply. Thus, therapy becomes part of the problem rather than part of the solution.

This dynamic is often, although certainly not always, at work in cases of therapy which drag on for years and years for no justifiable reason, where the same issues seem to resurface while no observable changes in the client's outlook or behavior take place. In extreme cases a therapist and his client will even engage in sexual relations. The client—while perhaps feeling some genuine sexual attraction to the therapist—goes along with the sexual encounter as a means of complying with the therapist's needs. While moral condemnation of such cases is easy, understanding its causes is no less important. The advocacy-oriented therapist, who does not appear to recognize where the therapeutic alliance ends and a different kind of relationship begins, remains the most likely type of therapist to allow such unprofessional conduct to occur.

How can the prospective or actual psychotherapy client evaluate whether or not his therapist is advocacy-oriented? This task can prove difficult. The best criteria are the seven factors of good therapy in chapter one. If a therapist provides feedback without superficial advice, if she helps the client separate facts from feelings with the use of reason and logic, if she takes a systems perspective, if she helps the client integrate the past into the present rather than simply rehash the former, then the therapist is surely competent.

Advocacy-oriented therapists, aside from showing an eagerness to become legally, sexually, or otherwise inappropriately involved with a client, tend to be advice-oriented. They lecture their clients and have a poor sense of personal boundaries. Many advocacy-oriented therapists remain angry about their own childhoods.

Consider the example of the therapist sexually victimized as a child. Although aware that she has angry feelings over the abuse, she does not yet know how to place her feelings in perspective. Unable to integrate the past and the present, she still thinks of herself as a victim.

Such a therapist may, consciously or not, encourage the client to conclude that she also was sexually abused—even without sufficient evidence to validate this claim. She might suggest that a client's dream about giving birth to her father's baby, for example, represents proof that the client experienced sexual abuse by her father, even in the absence of other evidence. Consequently, the client's relationship with her father deteriorates, and neither client nor father understands why.

No harm results from a rational agenda on the part of a therapist. A rational agenda does not interfere with assessing all of the facts in a logical, calm, and objective way. Understandably, many psychotherapy clients sometimes find it difficult to look at their lives rationally. Nevertheless, no excuse exists for a therapist to create more problems for a client by leaping to emotional conclusions. If a therapist seems more eager than a client to find evidence of a problem in the client's childhood, without sufficient proof, such a therapist may operate with an irrational agenda.

Even therapists who become legally involved with their clients are not necessarily helping them. Legal advocacy can destroy the therapeutic process and lead to angry, bitter feelings, especially if the client feels that the therapist does not do a good job for him in the courtroom. In one case, a man became bitterly disappointed when his therapist, who originally promised to testify for him as a character witness in child custody proceedings, suddenly decided not to testify after her lawyer advised her not to do so. Feeling hurt and betrayed, he subsequently terminated his therapy with her at a time when he needed help the most. While he made his own choice to end therapy, the therapist must accept responsibility for raising the client's hopes in the first place. The outcome could have been worse if the therapist had actually decided to testify for the client, since the client expected the same level of warmth, support, and encouragement on the witness stand as he had experienced in the therapeutic milieu.

I make it very clear to such clients in the beginning of therapy that I will not testify for them. I explain the nature of the therapeutic relationship and why such interaction outside of the therapy office is inappropriate and potentially harmful to both of us. When a couple prepares to engage in a custody battle, I tell them that psychotherapy is of no use. They have a choice: they can either settle their differences through the legal system, or they can attempt to do so through a conscientious process of psychotherapy and mediation. Attempts to do both at the same time almost always end in disaster, in my experience, usually because one (or both) spouses is simply playing games on the advice of his or her attorney.

A related problem involves the use of a psychotherapist as an expert witness. For the most part, asking a therapist to serve as an expert witness credits the field of psychology with more objective knowledge than it actually deserves. Judges and attorneys tend to inappropriately grant scientific status to psychotherapy. Even worse, psychotherapists who market their claimed credentials (e.g., expertise on "the disease of shopping addiction") as objective credentials are able to assert opinion as fact and get away with it.

While there is probably no danger in having a rational and honest therapist testify as an expert witness, I believe that therapists who are willing to fulfill such a role are much more likely to be advocacy-oriented. Advocacy-oriented therapists tend to have irrational personal agendas of their own, which will be reflected in their testimony.

Most judges and attorneys do not understand that the psychotherapeutic relationship should not be advocacy-oriented. Cynical attorneys often think that therapists view their clients the same way they view their own clients, as individuals for whom they are paid to advocate, regardless of the truth. Advocacy-oriented therapists, like too many attorneys, minimize the importance of pursuing the truth; but a good therapist is most certainly interested in the truth and would never wish to mislead the public into thinking he has knowledge he does not possess.

Judges and parole officers tend to view psychotherapy from one of two mistaken viewpoints. First, they see therapy as identical to medical treatment in which something is "done to" the client. They fail to understand the nature of free will, and do not see that therapy cannot occur without consent. Operating on this premise, they force a defendant into therapy. The defendant shows up in the therapist's office saying, "The judge told me I had to come here." Psychotherapy is impossible under such circumstances. Therapists do not have a metaphorical "bag" of treatments to perform on a client to somehow make him better. For psychotherapy to work, the client must feel uncoerced and be sincere about wanting to change. While the judge may actually be correct in stating that the defendant needs psychotherapy, the coercive element makes treatment virtually impossible. For this reason, court-ordered therapy is a sham.

The second error frequently made by judges and other court officials is their assumption that talking *alone* will somehow "cure" the moral and psychological problems of the convicted criminal. In cases of juvenile delinquency, for example, judges will suspend or lighten sentences if the family will go for counseling. Most judges fail to recognize that forcing families into therapy only makes matters worse. Not only are such families generally resentful about the referral and unmotivated for treatment, but they also have no respect for the judge because he did not sentence the delinquent harshly enough. Coerced families are hopeless psychotherapy candidates, in my experience. Family or individual counseling should not be a replacement for tough sentencing.

Sometimes, clients experience advocacy-oriented therapists as overbearing. A female client might feel unsure about her husband, who sometimes treats her kindly and at other times appears to be insensitive and harsh. Instead of encouraging the client to evaluate her marriage in clear, rational terms, the advocacy-oriented therapist might insist that the husband is not the right man for the client. The client may feel pushed by the therapist to make a particular decision (such as a separation). The client should let her therapist know when she feels hurried into decision-making. Good therapists will respect this concern and talk with the client about it. Advocacy-oriented therapists will continue to push, almost as if they have a vested, personal interest in the client's making a particular decision.

The best way to distinguish between a good therapist and an overzealous advocate is the degree of rationality the therapist displays. A rational therapist carefully observes each individual situation. An irrational therapist tends to look only for data which fit his or her previously formed conclusions. A therapist who thinks little of men, for instance, may encourage a female client to hastily conclude that her husband is having an affair. A therapist with a personal agenda because of his own negative experiences with alcohol may be quick to leap to the conclusion that the client needs Alcoholics Anonymous simply because she has a glass of wine with dinner each night.

The best way to avoid the clutches of an advocacy-oriented therapist consists of seeking out a therapist who views psychotherapy as a professional alliance, not a personal relationship.

Consequences of Past-Centered Therapy

Past-centered therapy rests on the premise that, the more insight and knowledge the client gains about his past, the better he can deal with the present. On a superficial level, this makes a lot of sense.

Even so, past-centered therapy and good therapy do not arise out of the same philosophy. Good therapists want to know about a client's childhood only to the extent that it interferes with the present. They understand that childhood factors can lead to the formation of irrational ideas and behaviors. In past-centered therapy, however, the client rarely understands the purpose for discussing his childhood. Clients should ask themselves and their therapists, "Am I discussing my childhood in order to learn something which will help me with my present problem?" If neither client nor therapist can provide a good answer to this question, then the therapy will soon degenerate into frustration and hopelessness.

Good therapy seeks to evaluate and change, as necessary, the way a client thinks. While childhood experiences do influence the way an individual thinks and feels in adulthood, discovering the origins of such experiences do not guarantee therapeutic success. A client does not need to know every detail about the first five years of her life in order to recognize that she relies too much on the opinions of others in evaluating her strengths and weaknesses. It is more important for the client to identify her subconscious, emotional conclusions. If she discovers they are mistaken, she can change them without delving into childhood memories.

Even more fundamentally, bad therapies rest on the theory of determinism. The theory of determinism means that individuals have no control over their destinies. Their lives are determined by God, their parents, their ancestors, their genes, their gender, or by historical forces—everything except their individual reasoning abilities. A rational approach, while rejecting determinism, does not rule out the key influences of parents, ancestors, genes and history. It merely points out that human beings also have the ability to think. What this means for individuals is that the healthiest and most productive human beings are the ones who use reason and logic in the most effective ways. The task of psychotherapy is to help individuals solve emotional problems through the use of logic and, in the process, teach them how much power they have over their lives when they act on reason instead of unexamined emotion.

While early childhood experiences can affect an individual deeply, the individual still has the capacity to change and overcome her problems through identifying and, if necessary, changing her deeply-held assumptions about many issues. Bad therapy assumes that individuals are hopeless victims of their past and can do nothing other than to recognize the damage and apply for psychologically handicapped status.

The contemporary trend toward relabeling errors in thinking and behavior as "diseases" represents the idea of determinism taken to its limit. The more individuals are taught that life is out of their control, the more they come to believe it. The more they come to believe it, the more impulsive, violent, and economically unproductive many people become. This fact has implications for society as well as for the psychotherapy client. As Stanton Peele has so eloquently written:

> We are in the process of rejecting the idea that people can be responsible for their behavior when they are in a bad mood. We often see that how we word things reflects how we experience them. What does it mean to call people "suicide victims" and to say others suffer from "alcohol abuse" rather than saying that they have killed themselves or abuse alcohol (or, better still, that they drink too much)? Misusing the language in these neo-Orwellian disease formulations is the surest sign that we are deceiving ourselves in preparation for living in a desolate social universe that we decry but cannot change.[9]

Although reason and logic are essential tools for combating determinism, bad therapists often dismiss them as simplistic and even authoritarian. Good therapists, on the contrary, see reason as the only possible antidote to authoritarianism. The human mind is capable of solving psychological problems through a process of reason and logic. Such a philosophy empowers individuals to take responsibility for their own lives and be their own authorities.

Notice that, in the last several decades, authoritarian bureaucrats and religious fundamentalists are wielding more power, as the theory of determinism has become more influential. This development is not a coincidence. The more dominant the ideas associated with determinism and bad therapy become, the more people will look toward outside authorities to solve their problems for them. The more dominant the ideas associated with rationality and good therapy become, the more individuals will become economically, socially, and morally self-sufficient. In a society where therapy is a dominant influence, it is critical that therapists rely on rational approaches.

Although many therapists claim that, in the abstract, they disagree with the philosophy of determinism, they continue to practice a form of therapy (e.g., past-centered) which rests upon that philosophy. They do not seem to understand the implications of their own approach.

In good therapy, the theoretical implications are clear. Emotional states are consequences of thought processes, and changes in thought processes can lead to changes in emotional states. Rational introspection, defined as reasoning with one's feelings and emotions, represents the means for changing one's emotional state. Since introspection is possible for virtually all people, determinists are wrong to view human beings as the helpless byproduct of external forces.

How can the therapy client avoid the trap of determinism, given the fact that so many therapists subscribe to it? If a client spends multiple sessions with his therapist focusing exclusively (or mostly) on his childhood, and he does not know why, then he ought to *ask.*

Quite frankly, a client should not continue with such a therapist unless she provides good reasons for discussing childhood in therapy. Good reasons include the following: searching for some ideas of how to solve current problems;

wanting to do an assessment to make sure no mistakes are made in helping the client deal with a current problem; or, needing to discover some mistaken generalizations or "core evaluations"[10] made in childhood so that they can be modified and overcome in the present. Core evaluations, as defined by psychologist Edith Packer, are basic conclusions, or bottom-line evaluations, that we all hold subconsciously and apply to ourselves, reality and other people. Examples of core evaluations include, "I am a bad person," or "People are such that sooner or later they will hurt me." In good therapy, discussions of the past are the exception rather than the rule; therapist and client discuss the past only within a specific context understood by each, such as the identification of core evaluations.

Bad or vague reasons for discussing the past might include: having to "work through" past issues before moving on in the present; needing to gain more insight; or getting in touch with one's "inner child."

None of these vaguely worded rationalizations constitute good reasons for discussing the past in psychotherapy, and they all beg for an answer to the following questions: What does "work through" mean? How am I to know when I have "worked through" the issues? And what "issues" are you referring to? For what purpose do I need to gain more insight? What will this insight help me do? What does getting "in touch" with my childhood self mean? How will I know when I'm in better touch—will you tell me or will I just know? About how long will the discovery of insight take? And, by the way, what exactly is an "inner child?"

The bottom-line for the consumer is as follows: If a therapist has not been able to persuade his client as to why she must talk at length about her childhood in therapy sessions, then probably no good reason exists for doing so. A client should not waste her time in such a process, even a "therapeutic" one, for which she sees no clear purpose.

Summary

The therapy novice should not become overwhelmed about all the potential hazards of participating in psychotherapy. Simply by using his head and the guidelines provided in this book, a prospective client has every chance of finding the right therapist. By holding himself responsible for finding a competent and rational therapist, the client is paving the way for making other important decisions in his life through the use of conscious principles and guidelines, as opposed to random emotional cues.

The consumer should ask himself the following question before his first session of therapy: "What am I hiring this therapist to do?" The individual ought to write down the answer to this question. He must have an idea of what he wants to see change and be able to identify his expectations as best as he can. If he is so emotionally distressed that he finds this task impossible, he can defer the process until the first session. A good therapist will assist in this process during a first session.

By now one should be able to see why bad therapy is *worse* than no therapy at all. One might also see the implication that a rational approach to life can prevent bad therapy from becoming harmful to one's long-term well-being. The next chapter provides more detail about what a rational approach to life actually involves.

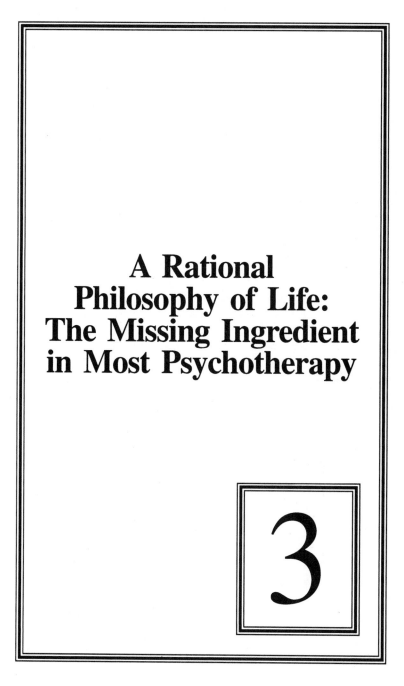

A Rational
Philosophy of Life:
The Missing Ingredient
in Most Psychotherapy

3

Good psychotherapy rests upon a rational philosophy of life.

A rational philosophy of life includes a basic recognition that feelings are not, by themselves, a means of identifying facts. Psychiatrist David Burns[11] puts it this way:

> Even though your depressing thoughts may be distorted, they nevertheless create a powerful illusion of truth.
>
> Let me expose the basis for the deception in blunt terms—your feelings are not facts! In fact, your feelings, per se, don't even count—except as a mirror of the way you are thinking.

Abnormal emotions, created by distorted thoughts, feel just as valid and realistic as legitimate emotions created by undistorted thoughts. People in emotional distress automatically attribute truth to their feelings and need help in recognizing that the feelings may not be valid.

Feelings, of course, can be valid. If you *feel* frightened by a major earthquake, for example, your evaluation relies upon the obviously correct assumption that major earthquakes do threaten your life. The central implication of Dr. Burns' point is that an *objective* reality exists independent of what one feels at a given moment: logic, rather than pure emotion, must be utilized in order to assess what the facts of reality are.

Another implication of Dr. Burns' point is that emotions are consequences of subconscious thoughts. In the words of Ayn Rand,

> Your subconscious mind is like a computer—more complex a computer than men can build—and its main function is the integration of your ideas. Who programs it?
>
> Your conscious mind. If you default, if you don't reach any firm convictions, your subconscious is programmed by chance—and you deliver yourself into the power of ideas you do not know you have accepted.
>
> But one way or the other, your computer gives you print-outs, daily and hourly, in the form of e*motions*—which are lightning-like estimates of the things around you, calculated according to your values. If you programmed your computer by conscious thinking, you know the nature of your values and emotions. If you didn't, you don't.[12]

In other words emotions are *caused* by one's subconscious thoughts, ideas or premises; these premises or ideas may be logical or they may be illogical. Since feelings are not necessarily facts, one must accept responsibility for identifying one's emotional "printouts" and checking whether or not such "lightning-like estimates" do indeed conform to reality.

While such a task often poses difficulty, it remains achievable with conscientious effort. For an individual, the failure to distinguish feelings from facts results in psychological chaos. As Leonard Peikoff points out,

> The ideas and value-judgments at the root of
> a feeling may be true or false; they may be
> the product of meticulous logic or of a
> slapdash mess; they may be upheld in ex-
> plicit terms, or they may be subconscious
> and unidentified.[13]

What happens when there is an apparent conflict between what one thinks and what one feels, between conscious thoughts and feelings created by subconscious
thoughts? Peikoff continues,

> When this occurs, the conscious ideas may
> be correct and the subconscious ones mis-
> taken. Or the reverse may be the case: a man
> may consciously uphold a mistaken idea
> while experiencing a feeling that clashes with
> it, one that derives from a true subconscious
> premise.[14]

Feelings are nothing more than subconscious, or *automatized,* thoughts. Automatized thoughts, as the name
implies, happen automatically or spontaneously. They occur outside of one's conscious, logical control.

Conscious thoughts, in contrast, derive from a process
of reason and logic, a process which, unlike emotions, is
voluntary and self-generated. The husband who reasons,
"My wife was late for our dinner appointment, but today
she picked up my dry cleaning without my asking her.
Clearly I can't say that she doesn't love me, or that she's
hopelessly inconsiderate," is engaging in a conscious, rational process of logic. The husband who physically strikes
his wife for lateness, however, operates on the subconscious
premise that "however my wife appears to me in this par-

ticular moment is how she *is*. I do not need to think further; my feelings are all I need."

In the first example, the husband implicitly takes responsibility for recognizing that a feeling of the moment and actual reality may be two different things; this is why he takes the time to use reason and logic to try and identify whether his negative feelings toward his wife represent fact or fiction. The man in the second example, by defaulting on the necessity of separating feelings from facts, subconsciously views an emotion as an adequate substitute for logic and reason. Even if he has never given any thought to such broad and abstract concepts as logic and reason, he has, nevertheless, to paraphrase Rand, delivered himself into the power of assumptions he does not realize he has.

While most people do not beat their spouses, all human beings need to rely on logic and reason in order to avoid acting impulsively or being unduly influenced by their emotions. To stop and analyze one's troubling emotions and determine to what extent, if any, they correspond to the facts can prove a difficult task.

Many individuals feel that they should not have to exert the effort of thinking and reasoning, especially for something so seemingly natural as acquiring a healthy psychological state. As clients sometimes say to me in therapy: "I don't want to think about this; I just want the bad feelings to go away!"

Yet if man is a *rational* animal as opposed to a merely instinctive animal, then what is the alternative? Recognizing that feelings do not always correspond to reality, and accepting the responsibility for figuring out what truly *is* the reality of a particular situation, form the essence of a rational philosophy of life. Good psychotherapy must help human beings learn how to place reason and logic above unexamined feelings. In so doing, good therapy helps them live in accordance with their nature as rational animals.

Do I Go With My Feelings or My Head?

There does not have to be any prolonged psychological warfare between thoughts and emotions. If the thoughts underlying one's emotions are illogical, they are capable of being modified so that the emotions will no longer be experienced as frequently or as intensively (if at all). If the thoughts underlying one's emotions are valid, then one is free to enjoy the emotions to the fullest extent.

Consider a highly simplified example.

If a man enters a home with a gun and points it squarely at his victim's forehead just above the eyes, the victim quite naturally experiences a range of initial emotions including shock, horror and terrified disbelief. Such feelings rely upon the subconscious premises that (1) the gunman is a serious criminal, (2) the gun is loaded and works properly, and (3) the man will shoot if he decides it is necessary or even if he merely feels the impulse to do so. Obviously, emotional reactions such as terror and horror are logical and appropriate under these conditions.

Now consider the same situation but in a different context. Imagine that it is Halloween, and the victim's next door neighbor telephones him shortly before the gunman's arrival to inform him that a mutual friend will be showing up with a mask and gun as a prank. When the "gunman" arrives, the "victim" naturally does not experience terror; his neighbor's warning provided him with a different evaluation of the man's intentions and identity than would have been the case in the absence of such a warning. If the victim evaluates the gunman as a serious criminal, the emotional printout reads: *terror.* If the victim evaluates the man as a friend in disguise playing a harmless prank, the emotional printout reads: *humor.*

Although most of life does not involve such unusual examples, the general principle applies to all human situations. Furthermore, feelings, because they are subconscious and automatized, do not imply the same level of responsibility as conscious thinking. Feelings resemble spilled milk: why cry over them or try to repress them once they have occurred? Repressing, denying or evading does not make feelings go away; it simply provides an excuse for not discovering their true causes. Feelings by themselves enjoy no moral status and should not in this sense be judged as "good" or "bad"; only the underlying thought or premise can be judged as logical, illogical, or some combination of the two.

Clients, in my experience, sometimes do not fully understand this distinction. Often individuals grow up in emotionally repressed environments and learn, quite mistakenly, that one can think "bad thoughts" or have "bad feelings." In recent decades there has quite appropriately been a great deal of rebellion against such psychologically restrictive environments and the damage they can cause to one's self-esteem.

While feelings alone enjoy no moral status, the underlying assumptions upon which they rely can be correct or mistaken. *Reasoning* with one's feelings emerges as the alternative to either repressing them or blindly following them.

Feelings can provide clues to understanding how one really thinks. A feeling of envy and hatred at the success of a friend, for example, reveals a belief that one person's gain represents another person's loss. A feeling of intense rage when a computer does not do what it is expected to do, for example, suggests that inanimate objects have free will and are therefore capable of unreasonable, unjust actions. A feeling of joy and pride upon the completion of a long-term goal, such as a medical degree or a work of art, suggests that the individual gives himself credit for his accomplishment and evaluates it as something good.

All feelings result from a corresponding and underlying thought or idea, even if that thought is not immediately or easily accessible to the individual. One should first identify the feeling so it may then be scrutinized as necessary to determine if the thought which caused it can withstand logical scrutiny. This process, known as rational introspection, is the subject of a later discussion. For now, it is helpful to keep these basic ideas in mind:

Feelings:
1. are outside of one's immediate control;
2. are automatic;
3. develop subconsciously, from implicitly held ideas and assumptions;
4. cannot be directly changed—only indirectly (through logic and reason);
5. happen effortlessly.

Thoughts:
1. are within one's immediate control, whenever one chooses to focus on them;
2. are voluntarily induced, and can never be forced;
3. develop consciously, in the form of explicitly reasoned ideas and assumptions;
4. can be directly changed—through a process of logic and reason;
5. require effort.

Lesson:
Change, as necessary, the illogical thoughts and assumptions. Let the feelings take care of themselves.

The Repressor versus the Emotionalist

Everyone must understand the basic distinction between thoughts and feelings in order to avoid mental disorders or chronic unhappiness. If a person rejects the view that feelings are simply automatized thoughts or fails to understand it fully, then he sets himself up for psychological problems. He will see himself as incapable of changing his feelings, and as a result he will go in one of two destructive psychological directions, each summarized by the following statements: (1) "Since I cannot control my feelings, I must ignore them and never acknowledge them to myself or others" (the repressed view); or (2) "Since I cannot control my feelings, I should simply accept them and use them as guides to thought and action" (the emotionalist view). Each view has psychological and social implications.

The repressed view involves excessive restraint and rigidity; it may take the form of a nostalgic longing to return to the "good ol' days" before there were psychotherapists— when individuals did not pay so much attention to their feelings and simply *endured* life instead. In the realm of parenting and child discipline, to spare the rod was to spoil the child. Child abuse was not seriously recognized and studied. Families held together, even in the midst of sexual and physical abuse, and a creed of duty and obligation took priority over personal self-fulfillment. Church officials set often arbitrary rules, inconsistently followed and rarely questioned. Everything seemed so simple. Feelings represented inconveniences at best, and immoral transgressions at worst. Children learned about the danger of "impure" or "bad" thoughts and held themselves responsible for random feelings just as they did conscious actions. On a superficial level, life seemed better and happier. In reality, many individuals suffered from a profound degree of emotional repression, denial and self-hatred.

The emotionalist view, on the other hand, is permissive and feeling-centered. It may take the form of a conviction that since the repressed view often leads to dishonesty, unhappiness and hypocrisy, the only alternative is to live solely by one's momentary urges and feelings. While such a view initially holds great appeal to an individual or a society previously operating under the repressed view, over a period of time its damaging consequences become apparent. The emotionalist view, like a speeding train approaching a brick wall at an ever-accelerating pace, inevitably collides with the raw truth that feelings do not always correspond to the facts.

A life lived on impulse and pure emotion can lead to arguably worse disasters than repression. A life lived on sexual impulse, for example, leads to a callously cynical view of romantic love. Traditional and invaluable support systems such as families begin to collapse under the weight of widespread divorce and grossly mistaken ideas about how to raise children properly. Nostalgia for the "good ol' days" of self-imposed repression emerges, and social conservatives snarl, "See? I told you so! Forget about your feelings. We must return to the good old days of repression, before there were psychotherapists and all these other liberal kooks who don't know what they're doing. The old way is the right way." Such people conveniently overlook the fact that the old way helped create the current disaster.

Does any of this sound familiar?

Both the permissive and repressive views have *some* good points to make. Permissive thinkers are correct that emotional repression is simply an unacceptable and impossible way to live. At the same time, repressive thinkers are correct that a life lived by emotionalism is equally, if not more, destructive in the long-run. However, each view shares a mistaken premise: that no alternative to repression or emotionalism exists; an individual must choose one or the other and settle for it as the lesser of two evils since human nature is fundamentally flawed anyway. Each view ignores the possibility of an alternative based upon reason, psychological independence, and conscious self-awareness.

Contrary to this false dichotomy, a rational philosophy of life does not mean a rejection of emotions; it simply means a rejection or emotions as necessarily equivalent to facts and appropriate guides of action. The rational individual listens to his emotions without feeling compelled to act immediately upon them. While he recognizes that he cannot wallow indefinitely in indecision, he also understands that no decisions (especially important ones) can be made without careful and logical consideration. The rational individual holds a long-term perspective even as he lives each moment of his life to the fullest extent possible. The only restraint he imposes on himself is to examine his feelings carefully and try not to act on them unless or until he is logically convinced such feelings are valid.

With respect to social relationships the rational individual also acts in his own objective self-interest. A rational and psychologically healthy individual cares more about his own life, his own possessions, and his own loved ones than those of the masses. Yet he also respects the rights of others to their own property as well as their right not to have his values or beliefs forcibly imposed on them. He does not cave in to the envy of those who hate him for his honestly achieved successes.

At the same time, he is generous and compassionate when he sees reason to be and when he is not acting under compulsion; he happily and guiltlessly pursues a policy of voluntary good will and kindness toward deserving others but resents any attempt to have such qualities forced on him. The central purpose of his life is productive work, not serving others. He consciously adopts realistic principles and holds firm to his convictions; he sees principles as eminently practical. He thinks long-range and does not sacrifice his ideals or creative ambitions to any shorter term desires for approval or gratification. At the same time, he rejects a puritanical work ethic in favor of a career that stimulates his mind and that he finds enjoyable in and of itself.

The rational man or woman consciously rejects both the permissive and repressive views in favor of the life-loving, long-range approach just described. Such an approach depends upon a proper understanding of the difference between thoughts and feelings, an understanding that leads over time to a harmony between thoughts and feelings as well as a corresponding sense of peace and self-confidence. Such a psychological state is possible for any man or woman willing to accept responsibility for replacing the mechanisms of repression and emotionalism with rational, life-loving self-interest.

Introspection

If neither repression nor emotionalism is healthy, then how can one become rational? If one has been a repressor or an emotionalist for so long, how can he change? A rational philosophy of life seems so obvious, yet is it really as easy as it sounds to become "rational?"

Absolutely not.

Becoming rational—and attempting to stay that way— is one of the hardest tasks a person will ever undertake. The fields of psychology and its parent discipline, philosophy, first need to convince people that they *ought* to strive for rationality. Complicating this task are the blatantly irrational influences of contemporary psychotherapies, many of which encourage emotionalism and scoff at reason. The fact remains that every individual human being must learn how to be rational from scratch, no matter what era or circumstances into which he is born. While the principles of rationality are relatively easy for an adult to comprehend on the theoretical level, putting them into practice in any consistent way can be extraordinarily difficult. The best way to develop rational habits is to learn and practice *introspection.*

Introspection refers to the self-monitoring of one's thoughts and feelings so that reason and logic can be applied to them. It is a cognitive, intellectual process directed inward, focusing on and identifying the internal processes of one's consciousness.[15] Introspection involves the willful and conscious attempt to (1) identify one's feelings about a given situation or event, and (2) take responsibility for assessing the relationship between those feelings and reality.

Philosophy, which concerns itself with generalized theories about human knowledge and the human mind, is the parent discipline of psychology. Philosopher Ayn Rand made the point that an emotion by itself tells an individual nothing about reality beyond the fact that something makes the individual feel something. Without a commitment to introspection, a person will not discover what he feels, what arouses the feeling, and whether his feeling is an appropriate response to the facts of reality. The two basic questions of the introspector are *"What* do I feel?" and *"Why* do I feel it?"[16]

In monitoring her thoughts and emotions, for example, a woman might identify the following feeling: "My husband does not love me."

Since such an emotion is naturally quite troubling to the woman, she must first assess its relationship to reality. The introspection process involves asking herself the following questions and answering them carefully and with as much time as she needs in order to do a thorough job.

1. What are the facts which support this conclusion, if any?

    a. He is frequently half-an-hour late for dinner.
    b. He sometimes forgets to kiss me on the way to work.
    c. He doesn't act enthused when I talk about my desire to start my own business.

2. Am I leaving out potential factors which might support a different conclusion? (Play the "devil's advocate." Assume for a moment your conclusion is wrong. What arguments can you offer against it?)

    a. He has a lot of responsibility at his job, which requires him to stay overtime; while he could probably be a little more considerate about calling me, it's hard to say this means he does not love me.
    b. He tends to get too wrapped up in his job. This makes him absent-minded about others in his life. While this is not necessarily an excuse, and I need to find effective ways to let him know this bothers me, it hardly means that he does not love me. After all, he is very affectionate on the weekends and our sex life is pretty good.
    c. While it is true that a loving husband does get excited about his wife's ambitions, his apparent lack of enthusiasm does not mean he does not care.

        Perhaps he is too preoccupied with his own job.

Or perhaps he is worried I will become more independent and leave him. While neither of these possible reasons are necessarily excuses, they may at least explain what is going on. I need to get more information about how he feels and thinks before I leap to the conclusion that he does not love me and seek ways to "punish" him.

3. Based upon the above, do I have sufficient data to support my emotional conclusion?

Clearly not. I can see that I need to rule out other explanations first. If I can honestly rule all of them out, then I might have a serious problem on my hands. But since there clearly is evidence that he loves me, the problems probably have more to do with preoccupation (on his part) and, perhaps, things on my part of which I am not aware. Whatever the story is, it is silly to conclude, from the available facts, that he does not love me.

4. What is the next logical step? (Therapists or friends can help with this portion of the exercise.)
Possibilities include:

   a. Bring the issue up to my husband.
   b. Suggest we seek a couples therapist for one session.
   c. Write a letter to him and ask him to give his reaction to me either verbally or in writing.
   d. Go out of my way to be nice to him for a week, and see if my conclusion is supported or weakened.

The opportunities for using the introspection technique are as numerous as the number of individual feelings one experiences in a given day. Most people need to introspect about serious emotional trauma or difficult decisions at various points in their lives, and the above introspection technique can ensure a rational approach to an emotional issue.

As a psychotherapist, I see the remains of much human tragedy and many broken dreams in my office. I often wonder how many futile love affairs could have been avoided or how many misunderstandings could have been easily solved in the beginning if only more individuals developed the habit of introspection. (For more examples of the introspection technique, see the appendix.)

Introspection requires application of a rational scientific process to the events of everyday life. Yet one need not be a scientist to practice it. "In his approach to external problems," writes psychiatrist Aaron Beck, "man is a practical scientist: He makes observations, sets up hypotheses, checks their validity, and eventually forms generalizations that will later serve as a guide for making rapid judgments of situations."[17]

Virtually all adult human beings have this capacity, if they choose to exercise it. Before rejecting this idea as simplistic or naive, one must vigorously question the widely held idea that "logic applies to science and abstract truths, but it has no applicability to daily life." As a psychotherapist, I cannot stress emphatically enough that nothing could be further from the truth. Introspection is within the power of virtually any individual who is willing to *think* about an issue instead of acting impulsively. If scientists, the professional introspectors, did not approach their work with caution, tenacity and rationality, there would never have been a vaccine for polio or any of the other technological achievements most of us take for granted. Everyone, not only scientists, needs to introspect in order to survive and psychologically flourish.

Remember that for everyone, scientist and non-scientist alike, the key word is *willing*. Contemporary psychology, as already pointed out, emphasizes the social and biological factors which supposedly determine human destiny. Left out of psychology's first century, however, was any recognition of the nature of human choice. Introspection and cognitive therapy introduce the philosophical principle of free will into the realm of psychotherapy. Relying upon the principle of free will, the psychotherapy client can come to terms with his basic nature as a rational, volitional being.

Implicitly or explicitly, the good cognitive psychotherapist encourages the client to address certain fundamental questions even though the focus of therapy may be on very concrete types of issues. For example: Given the physiological and social factors over which one has little or no immediate control, what *choices* do humans nevertheless have over their lives? How can individuals become more psychologically healthy regardless of the physical or social conditions into which they are born? What psychological factors allow the individual to rise above the conventional standards and other contextual factors in his midst if he so desires and chooses? What allows the human to reject standards or behaviors he sees as invalid, since he is not a lower animal and cannot count on preprogrammed biological instincts or guaranteed membership in the animal pack to guide him? These are important questions historically ignored by most psychotherapists.

Psychology and psychotherapy have yet to increase our knowledge about human choice because so far these fields have preoccupied themselves with the ideas of social and biological determinism. For this and other reasons, as some social critics correctly point out, the mental health profession seems to be turning Americans into a society of frightened, dependent creatures who increasingly cry out for social authorities to protect and take care of them. In reality, however, *bad* therapy creates certain negative trends in the mental health profession. A rational philosophy of life, rooted in the day-to-day habit of introspection, can gradually yet effectively turn things around for many individuals who currently feel helpless and depressed. Good therapy can help so long as one is just willing to think for himself.

Good psychotherapy has a role to play in the development of introspection. Therapy can serve as an educational tool to teach individuals not only how to introspect but also how to develop introspection as a habit of daily living. Once the process of introspection becomes habitual or automatized, the therapy client notices that she begins to approach emotional issues rationally as the *rule* rather than the *exception,* and with little or no coaching from her therapist. Although subtle and sometimes difficult to detect, the degree to which rational responses are automatized (i.e., happen spontaneously) is one very important and objective measure for evaluating progress in psychotherapy. Learning to *think* one's way through various emotional states, as opposed to acting on them or becoming paralyzed by them, must be a fundamental goal of any successful psychotherapy.

Integrated Rationality

I cannot overemphasize the point that *genuine* rationality does not involve the Mr. Spock-like repression of all emotions in favor of thoughts. To accept the view of man as a rational animal does not deny that emotions are both a normal, and potentially beautiful, dimension of human experience. A rational philosophy does not sacrifice emotions to thought, although to emotionalists it will seem this way. A healthy individual listens to her emotions and identifies them without prematurely concluding that they constitute facts. "Maybe this confusing emotion rests upon a fact," she says to herself, "or maybe it does not. Until I look at it logically, I cannot know for sure."

Both rational and irrational individuals *feel.* The distinctive feature of a psychologically healthy person is his habitual use of introspection to examine the truth or falsehood of his automatized thoughts (that is, his feelings).

Emotions are not worthless or somehow beneath rationality. So long as one has taken responsibility for checking the relationship of one's emotions to the facts, then one ought to be free to feel to the fullest extent possible. If an individual has objective evidence of an injustice committed against her, for example, then her anger is entirely justified. If a mother reunites with her kidnapped child, then her joy is entirely appropriate. In fact, one would question the *rationality* of these individuals if they failed to experience the appropriate kinds of emotions.

Nor is it true that emotions must always be ignored. *Listening* to one's feelings and immediately accepting them as facts are not one and the same thing. Most individuals, for example, have at one time or another experienced a bad feeling about someone at an initial encounter. After meeting a new person, a man might notice a feeling of suspiciousness. After the individual leaves, he might say to himself: "What was it that made me suspicious about this man? The fact that he wore a black coat? That's silly. But I also noticed that he would not make eye contact with me. This seems a little strange, but it could mean many things, including the possibility that he's just very shy and uncomfortable. I will note this incident, but not worry about it any more for now. The issue is shelved."

Notice how the rational individual can *listen* to his feeling without drawing unwarranted conclusions from it. The emotionally repressed individual would never have given himself a chance to dismiss—or even to shelve—the feeling of suspicion about the man. The thought, "this man is suspicious" would have stayed within his subconscious mind, unchallenged and unexamined.

The repressed individual equates rationality with the supposed absence of feelings. He fails to appreciate the inevitability of feelings. Psychologically, to be rational refers to the successful integration of one's thoughts and emotions. In other words, psychological health means the condition in which both one's thoughts *and* emotions correspond to reality. The typical benefits of such an integration include calmness, unconflicted emotions and a generally uninterrupted sense of peace and self-confidence. Repressors do not experience these benefits.

Just as repressors assume they cannot listen to their feelings, they also tend to assume they cannot risk showing their feelings to others—even loved ones. Emotionalists love to point out that "rational" (meaning: repressed) individuals are unable to cry or who show their feelings. Some feminist psychotherapists turn this into a gender issue, insisting that men are, by nature, "too rational" and women are, by nature, "sensitive, compassionate and caring," as if the latter qualities were the only ones desirable for either men or women.

Such critics fail to recognize that one cannot choose between thoughts and feelings. Yet both emotionalists and repressors attempt to make such an impossible choice. Emotionalists choose emotion over thought; repressors choose thought over emotions. Neither seems to recognize that thoughts and feelings must be *integrated,* not separated. To integrate emotions is to allow oneself to feel emotions, but also to rationally evaluate them against the facts of the objective world.

The truly rational—or integrated—individual has every reason to feel comfortable showing her emotions under appropriate circumstances. She has already checked the basis for her emotions. She wants to make her thoughts conform to reality—*not* make reality conform to her thoughts. She welcomes a challenge to her thoughts if it might lead to new discoveries about herself, those she cares about, or the world in which she lives. She allows herself to feel angry or distressed if what she cares about has been assaulted; she also lets herself feel joyful and proud if what she cares about has been achieved. Because she introspects as a matter of habit, she remains unlikely to experience chronic problems with out-of-context, troubling emotions. If she does, she will benefit from the help of a good psychotherapist and not view the need for such help as a reflection of character defects or weakness.

Reason versus Rationalization

Good therapy operates on the premise that *human reason* is the best method for solving psychological problems.

Human reason refers to the process of using one's capacity for both sensation-perception (sight, smell, taste, hearing, and touch) and abstract conceptualization (logic, inference, generalization) to form judgments and conclusions. While as human beings we share many biological characteristics with higher animals, the capacity to reason and judge remains the unique faculty of man—the rational animal.

Psychologically speaking, reason involves the voluntary, self-generated mental process required to answer the challenge: "Prove it." A chronically depressed or over-anxious individual, for example, feels horrified if asked to *prove* that life is hopeless. "Why should I have to prove it?"

he asks indignantly. "It's true because I feel it." Such an attitude represents the essence of irrationality—and psychological disturbance—no matter who the individual or what status he enjoys in society. The severely depressed individual is simply more honest about it than most.

Rationalization, on the other hand, is a process which might sound like reason but merely amounts to a phony imitation. "My wife has her many hobbies," says the man who plans to have a secret love affair, "so why can't I have just one hobby on the side?" Such a statement sounds superficially logical because of the way he phrases it; but he leaves out critical data. First of all, what are his wife's hobbies? If they are sewing and tennis, for example, how does he defend the fact that they are in the same category as sex? And what about the fact that he must hide his "hobby" in order to get away with it while his wife does not have to do so? What will happen to his sense of independence and basic self-esteem? And what about the obligation to his wife, given their legal and moral contract, to be honest about the affair if he thinks he should have one, so that she can at least be aware of the fact and decide for herself how she wishes to handle it? In such a situation, the man clearly ignores key factors which might lead him to a different conclusion; his rationalization prevents him from looking at those rather obvious factors. Were he to engage in a process of honest introspection, he would have to confront these factors and abandon his rationalization altogether.

Another example of rationalization: "I can steal money from my boss's safe. He has plenty of money. Besides, he does not know how hard I work when he's not here." It sounds logical enough to the rationalizer. But once again, an honest and thorough process of introspection can serve as an antidote to rationalization. The following factors in this situation merit consideration: (1) If it is OK for someone to steal based upon need, then it has to be OK for a criminal to steal someone's television set because he is poor and disadvantaged. Yet if the police refuse to pursue the criminal who stole a television because of such a principle, the owner of the TV would naturally consider this an outrageous injustice. How can this contradiction be justified? (2) The boss, in this case, owns the business in which the employee works. It is his private property just like the employee's house and car are his or her own private property. How much money the boss or employee makes is irrelevant to the issue of private, legal property rights. If the employee believes the boss is unfair, he can request a raise. He can take a new job, or politely threaten to do so and hope to get his boss's attention. Perhaps the employee could even start his own business, but it makes no sense to view his boss's success as a violation of anyone's rights. Only a rationalization, a form of pseudo-logic based on emotional convenience rather than hard facts, could allow the employee to evade either of these crucial points.

As these examples illustrate, rationalization and reason are fundamentally different in that rationalization cannot withstand the rigorous questioning of honest introspection— except through the creation of *more* rationalizations and evasions. The dead end of any rationalization is, "Well, I just know it's true because I feel it," or, "It's true because I say so." Reason, on the other hand, can withstand such criticism.

Many psychotherapists deliberately try to blur the distinction between genuine reason and rationalization. If a client develops a logical argument for making a particular decision or assessing a certain situation, the therapist might tell her, "You're rationalizing. I hear what you think. I want to know what you feel." This erroneous view has become so widespread that I frequently encounter clients who, when confronted with a cognitive approach to psychotherapy, accuse me of teaching them how to "rationalize." One must understand that honest introspection does *not* consist of rationalizing. Rationalization involves the sometimes willful and sometimes subconscious refusal to examine factors which might lead one to a different conclusion. Consciously or subconsciously, it serves as a means of lowering the anxiety one feels when not sufficiently in touch with the facts. The honest introspector, on the other hand, very much *wants* to consider all the facts, even ones which may feel uncomfortable or inconsistent with one's initial "gut" reaction. He understands that only through such a process can he hope to solve his emotional problem or dilemma.

To summarize, reason includes a process of introspection, an honest and thorough examination of the relationship between one's feelings and all of the facts one can access. Rationalizers make no such attempt to introspect about their emotions; rationalization, in fact, enables one to feel good about *not* introspecting in the first place. By its very nature, rationalization allows the rationalizer to evade or deny the need to introspect about an important life event.

My emphasis on reason runs counter to the mainstream view of the psychotherapeutic profession that unconditional acceptance of feelings, *with little or no reference to the facts of objective reality,* constitutes the essence of mental health. I reject the Freudian notion that man is doomed to act on impulse despite his better judgment. I do not think it repressive or chauvinistic to recognize that genuine rationality represents the healthiest way for individuals and societies to function. It *is* possible to place facts above "instinct" without turning into a miserable and repressed individual, despite what the emotionalist psychotherapeutic establishment insists.

In seeking to solve any emotional or life problem, the essential question is not whether one is being "too rational." The essential question is whether or not one's thoughts correspond to the facts. And only human reason, which includes a process of thorough and honest introspection, can lead one to the truth.

The Subjective Therapist versus the Objective Therapist

The introspective approach completely differs from that of the subjectivist psychotherapist who has traditionally dominated the mental health profession. Subjectivism refers to the psychological/philosophical view that no effective means exists for reconciling the events *inside* one's consciousness (feelings) with the events *outside* one's consciousness (reality) and that feelings are, for all practical purposes, facts. Subjectivism stands in stark contrast to Ayn Rand's philosophy of Objectivism, which upholds the view that the active use of one's mind, through rational introspection, represents the proper and psychologically healthy method of *interaction* between one's consciousness and reality.[18]

The subjectivist therapist encourages his clients to start with their feelings, identify them, and then to simply *stop.* For example, a client says: "I feel attracted to this person—perhaps even in love with her. I must continue paying attention to my feelings so I'll know what to do." The therapist may respond to this kind of statement with either silence or a nod of agreement. Therapists who leave out rational introspection—the *thinking* part of "working through" one's feelings—actually hamper psychological growth rather than accelerate it. No psychotherapy should encourage discussion of feelings *without any reference to the value judg-*

ments or underlying assumptions from which those feelings arise.

All individuals hold value judgments, consciously or subconsciously, and have no choice about this fact. The proof for this assertion lies in the fact that all conscious human beings experience emotions, which are nothing more than thoughts, convictions, and judgments in automatized form. "I like Joe," or "I am furious at my husband's reluctance to attend my sister's wedding," are both examples of automatized value judgments; the key is to discover what premises underlie the automatic value judgments.[19] The only choice an individual has is whether or not to make these value judgments conscious and explicit so that the judgments may be held up for critical, objective evaluation by oneself and/or others. Beware of the therapist who dismisses this process as too "judgmental." The subjectivist therapist who insists that it is wrong to judge oneself or others, even rationally and objectively, is himself making a *value judgment* that all value judgments are wrong.

What distinguishes the subjectivist therapist from the good therapist is that the good therapist either knows—or at least attempts to discover—the content of her own value judgments, and guides her clients in doing the same. The fraudulent nature of subjectivism lies in the fact that it enables the individual to escape responsibility for holding his opinions up to judgment since subjectivism rests on the notion that no truly correct or incorrect method of assessing reality even exists. Sadly, most mental health professionals rely, often without fully realizing it, on subjectivist premises because many psychological theories are rooted in this philosophy. After all, if the therapist sees objective knowledge as impossible, then why on earth obtain psychotherapy in the first place?

Beyond Introspection

After introspection the next logical question emerges: what do I do with my feelings once I conclude, beyond a reasonable doubt, that they are irrational?

The answer: *let them go.*

Tell yourself: "This feeling does not correspond to the facts. I have already established this through introspection. The feelings no longer have any use for me and can only create problems from this point forward. If I saw a wall in front of me, I would not attempt to walk through it over and over again, knowing full well that it is a wall and will not go away simply because I want it to. So why attempt to ignore inescapable facts simply because I do not like them? Why not spend my time and energy on things over which I do have the control to change?"

Letting go, of course, is much easier said than done. It can take anywhere from a few days to a few years to let go of an irrational feeling, *even if one already knows the underlying logical error.* Feelings are notoriously slow in catching up with the logical mind. The skill and expertise of the psychotherapist lies in his or her ability to find creative, effective methods for helping clients let go.

Here are several methods to assist in letting go of irrational thoughts.

1. *Reinforce rational ideas in favor of irrational ones wherever possible.* A number of methods exist for such reinforcement. Good therapy is one possibility. Another involves keeping a daily journal of one's thoughts and feelings, both as a way of avoiding emotional repression and developing the habit of rational introspection.

It is also helpful to identify behaviors and settings where one could become vulnerable to irrationality, as well as behaviors and settings where one generally feels happy and content. It is best to spend as much time as possible in the rational settings, doing the rational behaviors.

For example, an alcoholic is better off spending time with healthy friends than with other alcoholics. An anxious man is well-advised to spend time with calm, supportive people and to engage in activities he finds relaxing. A depressed woman ought to spend time with positive, successful friends as opposed to negative, gloomy people.

2. *Psychological entrepreneurism.* Try to develop and maintain a conscious belief that for every negative event in life, opportunities inevitably open up for new life challenges and experiences. An individual abandoned by her spouse finally has time for hobbies or career choices which might have been impossible before. If she loses a job, she now has a chance to try something different. If she has to move from the city to the country because of a job transfer, then she will encounter a way of life which has none of the disadvantages of city living and opens up the opportunity for new experiences.

It is, of course, absurd to pretend that absolutely every single negative event opens up new opportunities. But I think it can be stated with certainty that far, far more unrealized opportunities exist in life than most people realize. The person who develops the mentality of a psychological entrepreneur will—like an economic entrepreneur—always be looking for opportunities to meet needs which he previously did not know existed. Just as the inventors of Coca-Cola discovered a need for soft drinks which had previously been unknown, so can a psychological entrepreneur turn personal crisis and letdown into opportunity and creativity. A transfer to Montana, after having lived in New York City, provides one with a relief from crime, high taxes and dirty streets. A last child's graduation from high school provides a parent with an opportunity to travel, develop new interests and rearrange the house to suit only her own needs and preferences. I even know of a case where a relatively young client turned the death of a beloved romantic partner into an opportunity to develop better social and interpersonal skills, even as he grieved his devastating and irreplaceable loss.

Contrary to popular belief, entrepreneurism is not, by definition, exploitative, narcissistic, inhumane or destructive to the "social good." One need not run roughshod over the feelings and legitimate rights of others in order to take advantage of what life has to offer. In fact, as any individual seeks out and discovers new opportunities for himself, he is more likely to *help* others even though helping others is not his intention. If a woman decides to start a business, for example, the beneficiaries include those who find her product or service worthwhile as well as other individuals she may need to hire as employees. In becoming a psychological entrepreneur, the agenda involves always trying to find opportunities and pursue them rather than selflessly wallowing in negativity and helplessness.

3. *Discover the virtue of one's own independent judgment.* Rational individuals form their own conclusions and do not change them unless they see good reason to trust another's judgment (e.g., a physician, a car mechanic, an architect). At the same time, they make sure to base their own judgment on reason and introspection rather than raw impulse and emotion; this assurance enables them to stand by their judgment with confidence and conviction and only change their positions if persuaded by facts and logic. They are wise enough to understand that in order to enjoy the freedom of making individual choices, they must accept the increased responsibility which inevitably accompanies such freedom.

Standing by one's carefully thought out convictions represents the essence of self-esteem. A commitment to reason is the underlying cause of self-esteem, as opposed to the popular yet erroneous view that self-esteem arises out of unconditional love and fawning reassurances that one is right and wonderful and never mistaken. Self-esteem is impossible to obtain without confidence in one's ability to reason and, yes, accurately *judge* the individuals and situations one encounters. The better one's self-esteem and trust in one's own convictions, the easier it becomes to let go of irrational thoughts and intrusive self-doubt.

4. *Understand the nature of "reprogramming" oneself.* When a computer program is flawed in some way, the programmer makes sufficient changes in the program so that it works perfectly thereafter. In human beings the general principle is the same, but the actual process can be far more complex and time-consuming. Because human beings experience complex and often very powerful emotions, it may take many hundreds of individual instances of reprogramming before the new, rational idea becomes part of one's subconscious and automatic response system.

A person may conclude, for example, that it makes no sense to worry about the opinions of others. Yet she may have to "catch" herself in making this emotional error (in various situations) many times before the new, rational idea becomes her default, or habitual, automatic reaction. She will know that she has reached "default" status once she begins to *feel* the appropriate idea and not merely think it. Feelings are often slow to catch up with rational conclusions, but in the absence of internal contradictions they inevitably do catch up.

The computer analogy stems from the idea that all human feelings are consequences of subconscious thoughts. By changing or "reprogramming" irrational thoughts, an individual will eventually experience fewer troubling or conflicting emotions.

5. *Develop a time budget.* Many people discover that spending their time carefully and wisely reduces the intrusion of irrational thoughts and feelings, thereby assisting in the process of letting go. Most associate "budgets" with keeping track of finances and money. Equally if not more important, a time budget helps one keep track of everything he does. How a person spends his time ought to be treated with at least as much seriousness as how he spends his money. He ought to make use of every second—for work as well as relaxation and pleasure. An occasional inventory of one's activities can also prove useful. An individual can ask himself, "Am I getting adequate returns on my various investments of time? Are the friendships into which I invest my time rewarding to me?"

Examples of Introspection and "Letting Go" of the Irrational

Feeling: "I should go to the movies with Joe this evening."

Facts supporting this conclusion:

    (1) Joe is a nice friend, and I enjoy spending time with him;

    (2) I want to get out of the house—it's Friday night;

    (3) I enjoy the movie theater—the popcorn, etc.

    (4) Perhaps we can go dancing afterward.

Facts Which Might Support an Opposite Conclusion:

(1) While Joe is nice, he has this fascination for "blood-and-guts" films, and he flat out refuses to see any other kind. He will not compromise on this. I do not like these kinds of movies;

(2) I am trying to write a paper, and it would be good for me to spend some time on it this evening;

(3) I also need to get the house clean for my dinner guests tomorrow evening.

Based on the above, do I have sufficient data to support my emotional conclusion?

It's kind of a tough call. I really want to get out of the house. But getting the house clean and working on my paper are really important. And two hours is a lot to waste on a movie I am certain I will hate. Plus, if Joe is such a good friend, why does he not ever compromise on the type of movies he sees? Do I really want to spend so much time with a guy who actually likes such trash? He may have other qualities that redeem him, but why participate in this negative one? I have to say "no." The reasons for not going are stronger, and more important ones, than my reasons for wanting to go.

Rational Course(s) of Action:

1. Turn Joe down.
2. Work on my paper this evening.
3. Suggest to him that we go dancing or out for late-night dessert.

Methods for "Letting Go" of Irrational Conclusion:

1. Reinforce the fact in my mind that my reasons for not going are more important than reasons in favor of going. Fight the feelings that conflict with what I have already determined, through introspection, is the rational approach.
2. Psychological entrepreneurism—even though I am spending Friday night alone, I am seizing the opportunity to move forward on my paper and have the house clean for tomorrow's guests. I am viewing a potential negative as a positive.
3. Economy of time—treat my time the same way I treat my money. I will not throw it away on seeing a movie I am certain I will hate. It's two hours of short time on earth wasted. This strengthens the logic of my decision.

Feeling: "I should leave my wife."

Facts Supporting this Conclusion:

(1) We have little habits that get on each others' nerves.
(2) Many of our friends are divorcing—could it be that she and I are postponing the inevitable?
(3) We sometimes argue about silly things.

Facts Which Might Support an Opposite Conclusion:

(1) We are compatible; we have a lot of the same interests, like to go to bed at the same time, like the same type of food, sense of humor, etc.
(2) We have two teenage children we are raising together. It is disruptive to interrupt this process.

(3)   We share the same basic value system—family life, honesty, trust, hard work, relaxation.
(4)   We are best friends.
(5)   Our sex life is good.

Based on the above, do I have sufficient data to support my emotional conclusion?

Not at all. My wife and I share all of our fundamental values, on top of the fact that we want to raise our children together. We are best friends as well as sexual partners. I think I am overly influenced by the fact that so many of our friends have been divorcing lately. But that has nothing to do with my wife and me. Even if they all should be divorcing, and really have made bad choices or outgrown each other, how does it follow that she and I must do the same? Maybe we're one of those rare couples who can be happy for life.

Rational Course(s) of Action:

1.   Stay together.
2.   Try to stop doing the things that get on her nerves since I obviously have much incentive to stay with her. Also, she may then return the favor by stopping her annoying habits. If I make the effort to stop, and disregard childish feelings that say "I won't stop until she changes," then I have more credibility to ask that she change later on.
3.   Seek out good self-help reading or some other source to help with the arguing and communication issues.

Methods for "Letting Go" of Irrational Conclusion:

1. Discover the virtue of independent judgment—do not let the fact that many of our friends are divorcing, and saying how wonderful it is to be single again, influence my own judgment about my own marriage. The goal of life is to be happy, not to conform. I am basically happy in my marriage, and minor improvements will make me even happier.

2. Seek out new friends who have happy marriages. Include such individuals in my life in addition to single persons. If it is hard to find friends, then look for articles, movies and novels which portray happy marriages in fictional yet still realistic form. It will help remind me that happiness is possible, and not just a hallucination I must constantly question.

Feeling: I feel completely helpless and panic-stricken when it comes time to drive myself to work. I cannot explain it. It just overwhelms me. The freeway is so dangerous, and I'm so helpless!

Facts Supporting this Conclusion:

(1) Freeways can be dangerous places. Because of the high speed, accidents can be fatal.

(2) Because there are no traffic lights and many individuals travel faster than the legal speed limit, it is natural to feel uncomfortable at first.

(3) I am not used to freeways, so it is understandable that I will not like them at first.

Facts Which Might Support an Opposite Conclusion:

(1) The overwhelming majority of individuals who travel on freeways each day do not get into accidents. Many, perhaps most, accidents are preventable with just a little more caution. So long as I am cautious, I am almost never in imminent danger when I'm on the road.

(2) I can drive on other roads with some comfort; the same basic principles of driving apply to the freeway, only there are few, if any, stops.

(3) I control the car everywhere else; why can I not control the car on the freeway during the morning rush hour?

(4) I assume that my initial anxiety when getting onto the highway is abnormal, which leads me to feel panic. But I have no proof of this. Perhaps everybody has some anxiety at first, but I just let it overwhelm me.

(5) Panic implies an imminent, immediate and constant danger. But the facts contradict this. My own eyes tell me otherwise. Hours and hours go by without an accident.

(6) "Out of control" implies that the steering wheel and brakes do not work, and that I have no power to make them work. But my car does work, otherwise it would not run on any other roads either.

(7) Other people have no less incentive than myself to drive carefully, since they want to live too.

Based on the above, do I have sufficient data to support my emotional conclusion?

No. My panic is based on the assumption of immediate and constant danger. But in reality there is no such danger. Otherwise, half the human population would have been wiped out by now because of freeway driving. Feelings are not facts. My feeling of panic is grossly out of touch with the reality of the situation.

Rational Course(s) of Action:

1. Learn to drive to work on my own because there is no danger, and I do have control.
2. Enlist the support of any individual with whom I feel comfortable to help with the situation.
3. Seek professional help for suggestions and reinforcement on how to use thought processes to overpower irrational emotions.
4. Be hard on myself in that I will continue to make myself drive no matter what. Be easier on myself in that I will take it slowly, practice as much as necessary, and rely on loved ones/ therapist for help. Do not belittle myself for this emotion, because this will only make matters worse. Simply try to work on changing the mistaken reactions, however long it takes.

Methods for "Letting Go" of Irrational Conclusion:

1. Seek the help of a good therapist to help me reinforce the fact that my feelings are not a means of assessing the immediate reality of a situation. A therapist can also help me develop a plan for gradually adjusting to the freeway; starting on Sundays, for example, with my husband in the passenger seat. Driving in the slow lane is another possibility. Also, keep a journal

to help reinforce the idea that knee-jerk emotional responses are not facts, and I have the choice to think differently about this situation, even if the emotions will try to convince me otherwise at first.

2. Psychological entrepreneurism—recognize the fact that my anxiety is a healthy thing. If I felt *no* anxiety when getting onto the freeway, for example, I would not be as cautious as I need to be in merging with the speeding traffic. So, anxiety is not the problem. It is just letting my anxiety get the better of me and turn into panic which is the problem. But I have an opportunity to learn how to use anxiety in a positive way rather than my habitual method of panic. Turn this negative experience of anxiety into a positive experience from which I can learn and grow, and almost certainly generalize to other areas of difficulty in my life.

3. Recognize that "reprogramming" takes time. At present, I operate on the assumption that my initial panic at getting on the freeway is warranted. It will take time and patient, consistent reinforcement for me to eventually get to the point where I can get on the freeway with ease. It will not be an overnight cure. It will be two-steps-forward, one-step-backward until getting on the freeway with ease will be the norm.

Feeling: Life is hopeless. I cannot see any resolution to the problems I am having. I will never be able to do anything. No matter how hard I try, things only get worse. I've tried everything. I am going to end my life. I know of an easy, painless way to do it. All I need is a good time to do it.

Facts Supporting this Conclusion:

(1) I have had some bad experiences lately. For example, a potential new client for my business changed his mind about contracting with me at the last minute.
(2) In the midst of this crisis with my business, my wife has left me.
(3) I have no emotional support in my life, which makes things especially hard right now. I have no other good friends or family to lean on.
(4) I do have a hard time sleeping at night, and feel like I have no energy, kind of like when one has the flu.
(5) Life has always felt like a struggle and a burden, even in the best of times.

Facts Which Might Support an Opposite Conclusion:

(1) Not all of my experiences have been bad luck. I did make some bad decisions as well. I had evidence that my business partner was stealing money, for example, and I chose to ignore it.
(2) Not all of my problems have really developed all at once. My marriage has been going badly for a long time. From the second year of our relationship, I had serious doubts as to whether I made the right choice. I refused my wife's repeated offers to see a marital therapist. I insisted nothing was wrong.

(3) I have felt this way, to some degree, for years, even when things are going well. It's only worse now because everything is going wrong.

(4) Although things are very hard right now, I have survived and ultimately beat hard times in the past. The key right now is to try and remember what helped me before so I can use the same approach with a more difficult problem now.

Based on the above, do I have sufficient data to support my emotional conclusion?

In all honesty, no. I cannot prove that life is hopeless until I prove that it is impossible to learn from one's mistakes and not make them again in similar future circumstances. And I know from past experience that it *is* possible to learn. Individuals with even greater problems than I have now have learned, so I must be able to as well. Also, not all of my problems are due to bad luck. I am not a helpless creature floating through space and time, solely determined by forces around me.

I have the ability to make choices—I always have and I always will. While this means accepting the hard reality that I am responsible for some of my current problems, it also means I have the power to learn from them and not make the same mistakes again, and perhaps, finally, live a happier life.

Rational Course(s) of Action:

1. Seek psychotherapeutic and psychiatric help to determine what steps need to be taken to ensure that I do not commit suicide.

2. Ask a therapist or other trusted person to help me learn how to keep these emotions from overwhelming and paralyzing me.

Methods for "Letting Go" of Irrational Conclusion:

1. Reinforcement of rational ideas in favor of irrational ones with the help of a good cognitive psychotherapist. Keep a journal, do assigned reading and other tasks suggested by the therapist to help me stay focused.
2. Learn economy of time—only spend time doing what I need to fulfill my hierarchy of priorities right now. Learn not to spend my time any more thoughtlessly than I would my money. Learn that relaxation and mental rest time is just as important to fulfilling my long-term goals as hard work and determination. One without the other will not work.
3. Learn psychological entrepreneurism. Continually remind myself of the fact that even though my life appears to be caving in at the moment, everything happened for specific reasons and I now have an unprecedented opportunity to change things for the better. Out of catastrophe can come enormous change, growth, and learning.

Further Comments on Introspection

Introspection often requires considerable reinforcement and effort. The last example of the suicidal and depressed individual, for example, is clearly quite serious and will certainly require extensive therapy to help reinforce the accurate ideas and weed out the many mistaken ones. There is no guarantee that introspection and letting go of disproved emotions will immediately change everything for the better, but adopting introspection as a conscious habit does ensure that one develops and maintains a healthier approach to life and prevents such gloomy states.

Others will feel that introspection requires too much work, with or without psychotherapy. Yet what is the alternative? If one feels emotionally troubled or conflicted, then the likelihood of finding distorted premises, conclusions and generalizations in one's subconscious increases. How else can one identify his underlying assumptions without a process of introspection or something similar? And how else can he change such assumptions without applying the methods of reason and logic? Is it better to continue feeling awful and failing at life instead of making the effort required to think? Is it better to let others take over and do his thinking for him, as too many therapists are more than happy to do?

Sometimes clients fear that introspection will make them cold and unfeeling. But how cold and unfeeling is it to continue to allow oneself to act on the basis of mistaken assumptions? Acting on mistaken assumptions merely reinforces the sense they are true, further crippling the person. A phobic's fear of bridges, for example, is intensified every single time he avoids a bridge by taking a longer route home.

As more therapists become trained in the theory and practice of introspection, psychotherapy will become more effective and begin to lose its reputation for doing nothing expensively. In the meantime, prospective psychotherapy clients are well advised to choose a psychotherapist carefully.

Twelve Steps Therapies:
The Missing
Thirteenth Step

4

T welve Steps therapies include the group and individual therapies which explicitly utilize the Twelve Steps of Alcoholics Anonymous.[20] Such therapies have undergone an explosive popularity in the last decade and are no longer confined to Alcoholics Anonymous. Twelve Steps therapies have expanded to include a host of other groups such as Al-Anon (for people affected by someone else's drinking); Narcotics Anonymous (for individuals addicted to drugs); Nar-Anon (for individuals affected by another's drug problem); Overeaters Anonymous (for people who eat too much); Adult Children of Alcoholics; Sex Addicts Anonymous (for people with compulsive sexual behavior); and Gamblers Anonymous (for compulsive gamblers). There are probably many more which I have left out since the Twelve Steps philosophy is being applied to an ever expanding range of psychological and behavioral problems.

In this chapter I will evaluate the Twelve Steps philosophy which serves as the basis for these therapies. Although the wording of the actual twelve steps varies across groups (sex addicts, drug addicts, etc.), for purposes of coherence I will limit myself to the Twelve Steps of Alcoholics Anonymous. But it remains true that the same *general* principles apply to all of the various Twelve Steps programs.

A "philosophy," in this context, refers to a set of non-contradictory principles with the explicit purpose of guiding an individual through life. In order to appropriately evaluate the Twelve Steps philosophy, one must seriously consider the following questions: (1) Are the steps logically consistent, or do they contradict one another? (2) What are the implications of each of the steps, and do they serve the long-term interest of the individual who seeks to practice them? (3) Are the steps clear and coherent, or vague and ill-defined? (4) How applicable are the steps to daily life?

The Twelve Steps Interpreted

Step One: *We admitted we were powerless over alcohol—that our lives had become unmanageable.* If we are all powerless, then why pursue therapy—including AA or any other Twelve Steps group? If an individual cannot control his own drinking, then how will he ever stop? Since he cannot stop on his own, who will stop it for him?

The AA advocate will respond that the first step simply means accepting the reality that one's life is a mess because of drinking. Fine. An acceptance of reality obviously represents a crucial first step toward resolving the problem. But how does it help the individual to see himself, at the outset, as powerless to do anything about it? Does not the very fact the individual showed up for the AA meeting voluntarily prove that he can make choices and therefore possesses free will? Free will and the AA concept of powerlessness appear hopelessly incompatible.

Step Two: *Came to believe that a Power greater than ourselves could restore us to sanity.* Now the addict sees who is *really* in charge. The "Power greater than ourselves" will stop the drinking for him. How? No clear answer ever emerges.

Melody Beattie, a strong Twelve Steps proponent, freely admits that the Twelve Steps philosophy is religion—and in the same breath denies it.[21] She claims that the Twelve Steps are "spiritual," not religious. At the same time, she asserts that a Higher Power governs the lives of people. What exactly is the difference between the traditional Judeo-Christian God and the Twelve Steps Higher Power? If no difference exists, why distance the Twelve Steps from religion? No explanation is offered for this sweeping philosophical and psychological assertion.

Religious people believe in a mystical power outside of reality; they call it God, Allah, or by any number of names. Beattie and other Twelve Steps advocates believe in a mystical power outside of reality; they call it a "Higher Power." Yet the AA member is led to assume, without justification, that the two concepts are fundamentally different.

Words and concepts are *not* the same thing.[22] Consider the concept "chair." Suppose we decided to stop calling them chairs and instead called them "seating devices." Would this linguistic alteration modify the fact that the concept remains the same, even if the *word* used to identify the concept has changed? Of course not. Yet Beattie—and other Twelve Steps philosophers—retain the concept God while simply changing the name to Higher Power. None of this would present a problem for the therapy consumer, except for the fact that many therapists use the Twelve Steps as the basis for the supposedly scientific, rational procedure of psychotherapy.

A spade needs to be called a spade. The contrast between Twelve Steps and science is dramatic. No science, not even psychology, allows the introduction of spiritual belief or faith as a substitution for either logical inference or concrete evidence. Because of this faith requirement, the vague and misleading reference to a Higher Power is confusing and even harmful to the recovering addict. Psychotherapy does not explicitly teach people to believe (or not believe) in God; this is a matter for religious/philosophical discussion. Psychotherapy is supposed to teach people how to better manage their emotional states and rationally solve interpersonal problems through individual, objective actions. Faith does not qualify as an objective action.

Step Three: *Made a decision to turn our will and our lives over to the care of God as we understood Him.* By this step the conscientious AA member has every reason to feel confused. First, Beattie and other Twelve Step followers tell him that AA is not about God and religion, but about a "Higher Power." Then the third step encourages him to think instead about God as he *understands* Him. In other words: God exists, but do not call him God. In fact, think only about the God of your understanding.

What exactly does this mean? In religious traditions, from the most primitive to the most modern, God (Allah, or whatever) is generally understood as an all-knowing, mystical entity outside of existence. Religions generally teach their followers what role this Higher Being plays in their lives and how they should attempt to relate to It—through prayer or self-sacrifice, for example.

On the other hand, the Twelve Steps simply say, in effect, "Believe in a Higher Power, but make it whatever you want it to be." Left unanswered are two important questions: (1) Is there room for an atheist or agnostic in the Twelve Steps philosophy? (2) What does belief in a Higher Power have to do with learning how to make better choices and cope with alcoholism in the real world, on planet Earth?

Even more relevant, psychologically, is AA's encouragement of substituting one addiction for another. Beattie openly acknowledges this: "I had turned my will and my life over to the care of alcohol and other drugs . . . " she writes. " . . . It was time to remove myself from anyone or anything's control *(including my own)* and place myself in the hands of an extraordinarily loving God."[23] [emphasis mine]

The underlying message implicit in Beattie's viewpoint amounts to the following: "In the past, you let alcohol control your life. Now let the Higher Power control your life. Continue having no control over your own life. You have no power. You have free will but hand it over to the Higher Power instead of trying to use it yourself. Do not consider the possibility that the root of your problem may be that you did not use your free will *properly.* The problem is that you are incapable of using your free will at all."

This is therapy? This will put individuals back in charge of their lives? It seems cruel to tell alcoholics, who often have lost control over their lives, that they must surrender power to an unreal being. Alcoholics, of all people, need to be persuaded that they can regain control of their lives through their own rational choices and acceptance of personal responsibility.

Furthermore, if the alcoholic is inherently powerless, and since he does not have direct access to the Higher Power, then he presumably must put his trust in one of the Higher Power's emissaries here on earth. In traditional religion, the priest or the minister supplied the power that the ordinary individual was thought to lack. In the Twelve Steps, there is no equivalent except for the support group or the psychotherapist. (AA "sponsors" who guide members through the program may also serve this function.)

The third step of AA involves a kind of public relations attempt to make religious faith palatable to the science of psychology. It has apparently succeeded, given its strong endorsement by the medical and mental health fields, even in the absence of any empirical evidence to justify such a status. In reality, nothing can change the fact that AA, insofar as it promotes the notion of a "Higher Power," consists of faith rather than reason. It makes no sense to change the traditional name "God" to "Higher Power" and then imply that to change the name is to change the concept. Even more important, an alcoholic (often the greatest of excuse-makers) does not and cannot benefit from adopting the belief that his life is determined by a mystical entity rather than by his own choices.

Step Four: *Made a searching and moral inventory of ourselves.* This step encourages the individual to become more introspective. It inspires the alcoholic to look inward. Beattie, for example, encourages alcoholics to abandon self-hatred and instead "look at our good qualities . . . examine the standards we judge ourselves by, choose those we believe to be appropriate, and disregard the rest."[24]

Beattie's point seems clear, except for her ambiguity surrounding the term "believe." How, for instance, does one choose the "standards" to be kept and the ones to be rejected? Through reason and logic—or through surrendering to a Higher Power?

Beattie, furthermore, correctly implies that addicts do not suffer from too much selfishness but from *too little* self-regard and self-esteem. The rational individual who does not suffer from addiction problems understands or at least senses that being moral consists of acting in his rational self-interest, and trusts the use of his own mind and conscious judgment as far superior to following commandments blindly or acting out of a constant sense of unexamined guilt.[25]

Consider how the use of reason and objective judgment pertains to the issue of guilt. In order to allow oneself to continue feeling guilty, one must first have established objective guilt. Selfless individuals, including addicts, suffer from an ill-defined sense that they are guilty simply by virtue of their existence; that they are morally guilty merely for being human. Perhaps the addict has absorbed certain religious teachings which see man as guilty of "original sin" and therefore unfit for great accomplishments or sustained happiness on earth; or perhaps he absorbed equally false claims that it is unkind or unegalitarian to stand above the crowd and excel in any way, even if one seeks to do so through honest effort. Or, the unearned guilt may have resulted from messages he received in childhood, accurately or inaccurately interpreted, that he was not wanted or valued and was a burden to his parents. Whatever the many possible causes, the identification and gradual elimination of unearned guilt serves as an essential component of good therapy.

It is to the credit of the Twelve Steps philosophy that this concept is granted a certain level of recognition.

Step Five: *Admitted to God, to ourselves, and to another human being the exact nature of our wrongs.* The fifth step helps an individual discover the self-sustaining virtue of honesty. Honesty is actually *selfish* because it serves one's self-interest. The healthy individual finds it stressful to be dishonest for any period of time; it also weakens one's self-esteem to create a breach between statements and actions, and usually proves embarrassing when one is "caught" lying over the long run. As for dishonest individuals who do not experience (or allow themselves to experience) guilt for violations of other individuals' rights, they nevertheless pay the price through the legal, moral and interpersonal constraints placed on dishonesty in any rational, civilized society.

Of course, it is not enough simply to become honest with one's therapist or Twelve Steps group. One must extend the principle of honesty to all of one's relationships, both personal and professional, in order to become healthy. The therapist or group serves merely as a crutch upon which the client may practice until he has mastered the skills of honesty enough to engage in them without the support of therapist or group. To those who view Twelve Steps as solution-oriented therapy, no problems occur with this requirement. But for those who simply develop an addiction to Alcoholics Anonymous in place of the alcohol, breaking away from the AA group meetings or therapy sessions can be an extremely difficult task (and may never actually occur).

Consider the case of Fred G. Fred has attended AA for seventeen years. He socializes with AA members, he sponsors new members just starting to work the program, and his life generally centers on the issue of alcoholism and recovery from it. The only aspect of his life outside of AA is his job. He spends most of his free time at AA meetings or on 24-hour call for newly recovering addicts.

Fred seeks the help of a therapist when he becomes depressed and lonely. He summarizes his emotional condition as follows: "I am tired of my whole life being centered on the absence of drinking; I want a life based on the *presence* of something, some incentive for stopping alcohol in the first place." Through a process of solution-oriented, cognitive therapy, Fred discovers that in his recovery period he has merely replaced one form of addiction for another; because of his preoccupation with the Twelve Steps movement he lacks career goals, a romantic relationship and a general sense of identity as a happy and unaddicted individual. His constant encouragement in the Twelve Steps program has helped him to ignore this important issue; his depression now forces him to face it.

Step Six: *Were entirely ready to have God remove all these defects of character.* Once again the conscientious Twelve Steps follower must completely surrender his capacity for thinking to a Higher Power.

Everything good about the Twelve Steps philosophy so far discussed rests on the premise that individual humans are capable of thinking, changing their assumptions, and consequently changing their lives. Learning to admit the nature of one's wrongs implies a voluntary change in the way one thinks and acts. Learning the practicality of honesty implies a voluntary change in the way one thinks and acts. Learning to abandon self-hatred implies a voluntary change in the way one thinks and acts.

Yet now, in Step Six, the AA member hears that *God* will do everything for him. Beattie, as an important spokesperson for the Twelve Steps movement, fails to provide any justification for this sweeping reversal. "We become willing to be changed and to cooperate in the process of change," she writes.[26] The word "cooperate" implies some kind of partnership is involved, presumably between the recovering addict and God. The nature of this relationship, however, remains quite vague.

Furthermore, a basic question remains unanswered in all of this. *Who* is responsible for making the changes required of the Twelve Steps? God? Or the recovering addict himself? Exactly how does a "partnership" between a mortal human and an omniscient Higher Power work? How does one know that the Higher Power does not control the whole process, even when the mortal human seems to contribute to it through the use of his own reasoning abilities? And by what standards, if not the human's, can the process be judged and evaluated? It cannot be the Higher Power's because the Higher Power, like a conventional God, does not have direct contact with the individual and therefore does not give the AA member His standards.

Religion tells the alcoholic that a relationship with a Higher Power will *somehow* provide him with the means for living a happy and healthy life. Reason tells him that the use of his own mind—in a cooperative relationship with other human minds in a free society—will provide him with the means for living a happy and healthy life on earth. The religious person relies upon God and His emissaries here on earth; the rational person relies upon his sense organs, his intelligence and the accumulation of human knowledge over the ages.

Yet the poor Twelve Steps person, left with a vaguely defined "God as you understand Him," does not know where to turn. On the one hand, he needs to use his intelligence and, by implication, a process of reason and introspection in order to conduct a moral inventory, learn the exact nature of his wrongs, and so forth. At the same time, he must surrender to a Higher Power who supposedly has control over everything, including his ability to stop drinking and change other "defects of character." What is the nature of this Higher Power? What are the guidelines or commandments this Power wants him to follow while living on earth? "Whatever you *understand* them to be," AA tells him.

The contradiction which again shows itself in the sixth step is not exclusively a philosophical issue. The psychological questions remain: "Who is in charge of my life? *Outside forces*—God, society, destiny, fate—or *myself?* If God runs my life, then how am I to understand how God wants me to live? If *I* run my life, then how am I to figure out on my own how I should live?" The consequences of failing to answer such questions can produce a variety of psychological symptoms, alcoholism among them.

Step Seven: *Humbly asked Him to remove our short-comings.* Once again a contradiction exists between allowing a Higher Power to "remove" one's shortcomings or taking responsibility for such a task through the use of conscious, rational choices. Either the individual removes his own shortcomings through a process of cognitive and behavioral change, or God removes them, through a process of mystical grace, prayer, or whatever. It makes no sense to try and have it both ways.

Step Eight: *Made a list of all persons we had harmed and became willing to make amends to them all.* The eighth step can prove very worthwhile, psychologically speaking, for several reasons: (1) the step rests on the assumption that addicts are responsible for their actions including, implicitly, the impact their addiction has on significant others; (2) the eighth step also rests on the assumption that a rational process exists for objectively assessing one's behavior, even in the presence of powerful emotions; (3) it encourages a rational philosophy of life by forcing one to recognize that actions in the past, which may have *felt* right at the moment, were not necessarily right or healthy.

The eighth step also requires an honest look at the idea of earned versus unearned guilt. Earned guilt involves taking responsibility for something which one directly caused. Unearned guilt consists of taking responsibility for something which one did *not* directly cause. Most people, and particularly most addicts, do not distinguish between "earned" and "unearned" guilt, at least not consciously.

On the surface this distinction might sound like common sense; and the distinction between earned and unearned guilt is certainly quite logical. Unfortunately, many influential and powerful cultural institutions (e.g., church, schools, government) are not always so logical, and a failure to think carefully about the issue of guilt can lead to psychological problems such as depression, anxiety and substance abuse.

A healthy understanding of guilt requires, first of all, an understanding about the issue of responsibility. In my experience, the vast majority of individuals who are psychologically distressed tend to take too much responsibility for things they cannot control and too little responsibility for things they are able to control.

Alcoholics and other addicts are particularly guilty of this error. Individuals often drink alcohol in order to relieve stress in their lives, stress created by the mistaken assumption that they should be able to control everything. Instead of facing reality squarely and accepting facts, they resort to an artificial method geared toward changing their perceptions and perhaps even providing them with the temporary illusion that they can control everything, that they *are* invincible. While reality *feels* much better during the "drunk" phase, it still exists independently of consciousness and remains even harder to face once the hangover sets in.

Unfortunately, even though the eighth step raises important questions for the addict, it still does not explicitly define the role of unearned guilt in maintaining addiction. For this and other reasons, many of their followers end up in the therapy office, frustrated by AA for reasons they cannot understand and often fear to identify since AA is such a universally accepted method of treatment. If the addict can somehow infer the implication from the eighth step about the distinction between earned and unearned guilt, then he may gain tremendous psychological benefit from this stage of AA treatment. But in the more likely event he is unable to draw the necessary inferences, he continues floating in the clutches of his Higher Power.

A better way to conceive the eighth step, integrating rational concepts of guilt and introspection, might be this way: *"I used to assume that I could act on my feelings without first examining them. This led me to do many self-destructive things. Now I more fully understand that feelings are not necessarily facts. This requires me to think before I speak and act. It also places more responsibility on me for my actions. I can no longer say the equivalent of, 'The devil made me do it.' But it also means I have more power over my own life, to make myself happy and not have to live by anybody's standards except for my own."*

Step Nine: *Made direct amends to such people wherever possible except when to do so would injure them or others.* Like step eight, the ninth step implies responsibility for one's actions as well as a rational approach to morality.

Step Ten: *Continued to take personal inventory and when we were wrong, promptly admitted it.* The tenth step similarly encourages self-responsibility, honesty and introspection.

Step Eleven: *Sought through prayer and meditation to improve our conscious contact with God as we understood Him, praying only for knowledge of His will for us and the power to carry that out.* At least now the Twelve Steps participant has some vague idea—prayer—of how to make contact with his Higher Power. But, once again, how does surrendering one's rational capacity to a Higher Power actually help an alcoholic make better choices for himself?

Step Twelve: *Having had a spiritual awakening as the result of these steps, we tried to carry this message to others, and to practice these principles in all our affairs.* If "spiritual awakening" means increased understanding of how to make good choices and better use one's mental capacities, then who could disagree? Unfortunately, as we already know from the previous steps, "spiritual" most likely refers to a passive surrender to a Higher Power and a corresponding admission of helplessness.

The Facts about Alcoholics Anonymous (AA)

Popular perception is that AA works. Doctors recommend it. Therapists encourage it. Members of AA worship it. Journalists adore it. Politicians canonize it. Movie and television stars swear by it. Advocates for AA insist that no other method exists for treating the "disease" of alcoholism. Evidently no further clarification is required. A popular AA quote sums up the attitude of AA advocates quite well:

How do the Twelve Steps work?
They work just fine, thank you.

Whatever guides AA and the enormous amount of federal and private dollars that have been poured into it, an indepth understanding of its underlying philosophy is apparently not a top priority among its proponents.

In reality, available scientific evidence fails to support the enthusiastic claims of AA advocates. The conventional wisdom, as illustrated by the above quote, is that the successful "graduates" of AA are the best proof of its effectiveness. However, no scientific evidence supports AA's claim of much higher success rates than ordinary clinical treatment. According to researchers at the Downstate (New York) Medical Center Department of Psychiatry who take population differences into account, the data suggest that the success rate for AA participants is actually *lower* than non-AA participants. According to addictions expert Stanton

Peele, no study has ever found AA or its companion Twelve Steps programs to be superior to any other approach, including no treatment at all. Furthermore, addiction treatment approaches which have been actually demonstrated superior to AA in research have been consistently rejected by American government agencies which have a large role in funding and identifying effective treatment programs.[27] The reasons for this fact remain a mystery.

As already seen, a basic premise of Alcoholics Anonymous is that alcoholics are "powerless" over their addiction. Research experiments show, however, that alcoholics, rather than losing control of their drinking, actually *aim* for a desired state of consciousness when they drink. They drink to transform their emotions and their self-image. For alcoholics, drinking is a route to achieve feelings of power, sexual attractiveness, or control over unpleasant emotions. Alcoholics strive to attain a particular level of intoxication, one that they can describe before taking a drink. They are engaging in *goal-directed behavior* which suggests anything but powerlessness.[28]

The Case of Mr. L., an Alcoholic

Consider the case of Mr. L., who has difficulty controlling his drinking problem. He and his wife attend therapy on a weekly basis to develop better methods of communicating with each other. It becomes clear through the therapy sessions, however, that Mr. L.'s irrational frame of mind when he drinks alcohol is a major cause of the communication problems. When asked by the therapist to introspect about the feelings he experiences just prior to taking a drink, Mr. L. states, "I feel that my job is horrible and I feel like my wife is always on my back, and I simply want to be left alone. I just want a place to go and be by myself. There isn't any real place for me to go except the neighborhood bar. Crazy as it may sound, I go to the bar so I can escape my troubles and just not have to *think* anymore."

The case of Mr. L., a composite of many alcoholics and other addicts with whom I have worked in therapy, offers an excellent illustration of the point that such individuals consciously aim for a desired state of consciousness when they drink. I have never met an alcoholic who does not sooner or later admit, if he is honest and committed to improving himself, that he actively—albeit compulsively— seeks out the object of addiction. I am not implying that the alcoholic necessarily *wants* to be compulsive or to bring grief upon himself and others; but neither can it be claimed that the Mr. L.s of the world are victims of an insidious disease over which they have no conscious control.

In therapy, Mr. L. will need to introspect a great deal, and the therapist will need to challenge many of Mr. L.'s underlying assumptions including, just for starters: (1) the false belief that escaping to the bar represents the only logical alternative to dealing with his wife's complaints when rational communication strategies are available to him; (2) the illogical, adversarial belief that a contradiction exists between his own interest and his wife's interest, assuming that they really love each other and both want the same things out of life; and (3) the widely held but mistaken notion that "relaxation" has to consist of an activity without any thought or exertion, a viewpoint implicit in his desire "not to think anymore."

Given Mr. L.'s mistaken and irrational beliefs, it might be said that compulsive drinking characterizes the least of his problems, a mere consequence of holding erroneous beliefs. Given the specific content of these beliefs, the *last* message he needs to hear is that he is powerless over alcohol as

Alcoholics Anonymous will tell him upon his first visit to a meeting. In the short run the idea of powerlessness may seem reassuring and comforting to him, especially because his irrational beliefs have paralyzed him. But over the long run nothing can cure his alcoholism except a voluntary change in his approach to self-responsibility and self-interest.

More Facts About AA

Other research suggests that self-cure among alcoholics is much more common than AA advocates would have us believe. Untreated but recovered alcoholics, according to researcher Barry Tuchfeld, may constitute a "silent majority."[29]

Based on his research in Australia, psychiatrist Les Drew has described alcoholism as a "self-limiting" disease, one that creates pressures for its own cure even in the absence of mental health interventions.[30] Because alcoholism typically involves irresponsible behaviors, pressure gradually increases on the alcoholic to moderate or eliminate his drinking. The alcoholic may, for example, face losing his job or marriage unless he agrees to "sober up." While treatment may receive all the credit for curing the alcoholic, the alcoholic can only benefit from treatment if he chooses to engage in it. Pressure from loved ones and employers is often central to the alcoholic's motivation to change his behavior.

Spouses, parents or other loved ones of alcoholics often beg the therapist to "do something" to fix the problem, as if it were possible for a therapist to intervene without the addict's voluntary consent, just as an emergency medical technician intervenes at the scene of a car accident to save the victim. These loved ones soon discover that *they*, not the therapist, are the ones who have the power to create pressures in the addict's life (through refusing to run errands for him, refusing to pay his bills for him, refusing to take phone messages for him, refusing to lie for him, refusing to have sex with him, etc.). They have the power to make it easier for him to finally lower his defenses and admit that he, himself, needs to do something about his problem. And what if he still refuses to change his ways? Then the loved one may simply have to accept the addict as beyond redemption.

Unfortunately, individuals who overcome drinking problems on their own are not an organized and visible group such as Twelve Steps program members; yet most therapists, myself included, encounter such people on a regular basis. If certain individuals, whatever their number, can stop drinking on their own, then we already have proof that the Twelve Steps approach is not the only way to control one's drinking; other factors outside of having a formal support group, such as correcting mistaken beliefs and confused value systems, must be relevant to a cure.

Furthermore, how do we know that those who choose to stick with AA—and promote the program as successful— were not on their way to self-cure when they joined the program? As I frequently say to my clients at the start of therapy, "Making and keeping the first therapy appointment is more than half of therapy." Clients generally confirm the truth of this statement. A 1987 *Science* magazine study noted, in fact, that the best predictors of treatment outcome for alcoholics consist of the personality characteristics of the individuals who enter treatment, not the type of treatment itself.[31]

Research on AA and, by implication at least, other Twelve Steps programs using the same philosophy, does not back up the enthusiastic claims of its proponents. Increased analysis of the assumptions underlying the Twelve Steps philosophy will help explain why.

What's *Good* About the Twelve Steps Movement?

In reality, the Twelve Steps program represents a mixed philosophy. In other words, it contains principles which contradict one another. Consequently, it is impossible to reject the philosophy as a whole without at least acknowledging that many individual truths exist within it.

Twelve Steps advocate Melody Beattie has written a number of books (including the best-selling *Codependent No More*) which have done much to advance the movement in the last ten years. Included in her writings are three concepts influencing today's Twelve Steps movement. Viewed from a cognitive therapy perspective, these concepts are highly useful. These concepts are: (1) detachment, (2) "removing the victim," and (3) "undependence."

Beattie (1987) defines detachment by first defining *attachment*.[32] Attachment, according to Beattie, can take several forms:

> Becoming excessively worried about, and preoccupied with, a problem or person;
>
> Becoming obsessed with and controlling of the people and problems in our environment;
>
> Becoming reactionaries, instead of acting authentically of our own volition;
>
> Becoming emotionally dependent on the people around us;
>
> Becoming caretakers, rescuers or enablers to the people around us (firmly attaching ourselves to their need for us).

In a nutshell, unhealthy attachment involves sacrificing oneself to others for unstated, inexplicable or totally irrational reasons. Individuals in love with alcoholics and other addicts are particularly prone to attachment, according to Beattie. *De*tachment, in turn, involves a psychological reversal of this process through a change in one's views of independence, rationality and self-interest.

Consider the case of Mrs. L., the wife of the alcoholic who escapes to the bar to avoid his wife and the necessity of thinking. For years she put up with her husband's lack of support with the kids, his embarrassing statements in front of relatives when he was drunk, and his disappearance from the house when some sort of family or financial crisis required quick resolution. Why, the therapist asks her, did she so selflessly put up with these troubles for so many years?

Mrs. L. answers, "Part of the reason is financial; I don't have training for a good career, and my husband at least made enough money to pay the bills and keep a roof over our heads. But as I reflect further on it, part of the reason involves my expectations of a romantic relationship. I thought it wrong and selfish to ask that he address some of my concerns and act more responsibly around the house. I also got so used to his erratic behaviors that, after a while, I learned not to think about it so much. I would occasionally get angry, of course, but then he would go into a pout and I decided that he just needed more nurturing. I decided that if I nurtured him and loved him unconditionally, the problem would go away since he did not get enough of such love as a child. Instead, it got worse, and our fights became so frequent and intense that I finally called a therapist when I couldn't take it anymore."

Mrs. L.'s statement contains many implicit illogical beliefs, beliefs compatible with Beattie's idea of attachment. Mrs. L., first of all, assumes it bad to be "selfish" or, put another way, she sees it as inherently wrong to act in her self-interest. She probably took it for granted all those years that acting in her own self-interest would necessarily be acting *against* her husband's self-interest. But while such a mistake can be easy to make, if one thinks carefully, just the reverse is true.

If Mr. L.'s drinking was slowly destroying his chance to be happy and even to survive and contribute to the financial and emotional raising of his children, then how could it conflict with his self-interest to apply pressure on him to curb it? How did it serve Mr. L.'s interest, and therefore conflict with his wife's interest, to escape into a mind-numbing state and cheat himself out of the potential pleasure of kids that were happy to see him in the evening and a wife with whom he could become better friends and a more equal partner?

Even if the marriage was indeed a sad mistake, why not face the fact and arrange as amicable a divorce as possible so that everyone could move on with their lives, and the agony and addiction could cease? Only when Mrs. L. began to sense this contradiction, at least on some implicit, unexamined level, was she able to say "I'm fed up" and convince her husband of her determination to make a serious change.

The case of the alcoholic husband and the "codependent" Mrs. L., a classic one indeed, provides a good illustration of how subconscious beliefs and ideas determine behavior and emotions. The mistaken belief that self-sacrifice and selflessness equals love fuels the problem of codependence in the first place; only when both partners challenge and change this mistaken belief can they eradicate the dysfunction. Only when they realize that genuine lovers do *not* want sacrifices from their partners will they ever experience mature, fulfilling romantic love. Only when they are selfish enough to respect *themselves* will they be able to find a partner whom they can also respect and love.

"Removing the victim" is another Beattie concept utilized by many Twelve Steps therapists. In order to "remove" the victim, according to Beattie, one must eliminate the selfless habit of "caretaking" and "rescuing," as characterized by the following types of behaviors:

> Doing something we really don't want to do;
>
> Saying yes when we mean no;
>
> Doing something for someone although that person is capable of and should be doing it for him- or herself;
>
> Meeting people's needs without being asked and before we've agreed to do so;
>
> Doing more than a fair share of work after our help is requested;
>
> Consistently giving more than we receive in a particular situation;
>
> Fixing people's feelings;
>
> Doing people's thinking for them;
>
> Speaking for another person;
>
> Suffering people's consequences for them;
>
> Solving people's problems for them;
>
> Putting more interest and activity into a joint effort than the other person does;
>
> Not asking for what we want, need and desire.[33]

Most of these unhealthy behaviors stem from a more basic premise: "I owe my life to others. It is a virtue to sacrifice myself to others. If I'm losing or giving up something, I am being virtuous; if I'm gaining or acquiring happiness, I am being less than virtuous."

Such a belief system forces an individual to choose between what she sees as moral and what makes her happy. The happier she becomes, the more guilty she feels; the more miserable she feels, the more she assumes she is fulfilling her moral obligation to God or others. What a lousy choice! This moral-happy dichotomy has many psychological consequences, including chronic rage, resentment and mental exhaustion.

If one holds the assumption that he has an obligation to do the impossible, then he must feel guilty when failing at the impossible. At the same time, if he bangs his head against a wall long enough, he starts to get angry at the wall for causing his pain—all the while overlooking the fact that he need merely stop banging his head and the pain will stop. The same applies to individuals who are "codependent" or "rescuing" by Beattie's definition. I label such behavior *selflessness*. Selfless premises, in my experience, underlie many psychological problems. Correcting selfless premises is a crucial component of good therapy yet remains generally unacknowledged even by most cognitive therapists.

"Undependence" is a term cited by Beattie to describe "that desirable balance wherein we acknowledge and meet our healthy, natural needs for people and love, yet we don't become overly or harmfully dependent on them."[34] In other words, relationships and friendships do not simply require mutual need. Good relationships also depend upon trust and respect, especially for the sake of longevity. Love is *not* enough.

The unhealthiest relationships sacrifice respect to need; the concept of respect is barely even recognized in relationships with needy, selfless individuals.

An alcoholic husband, for example, needs a wife who will sanction his self-destruction by never mentioning it aloud; deep down the husband probably hates her because she refuses to stand up for herself and identify him as the troubled creature he is.

A woman with low self-confidence needs a husband who will obey the unwritten rule that he must never criticize her; deep down she probably despises her husband for being so patronizing and selfless, never having the nerve to hold her responsible for a standard of logic and common sense.

A man with a "pathological" need for control and domination needs a wife and children who will quietly submit to his arbitrary and irrational demands; deep down he probably senses how they fear him, and he hates them for it because, psychologically, he knows he is the weakest one of them all.

Unlike abusive husbands, healthy individuals *need* each other but not in the same respect as unhealthy ones. Healthy individuals experience need in the sense that they would rather have a healthy relationship than have none at all. But they do not fall into the trap of accepting *any* relationship as better than none at all.

Healthy individuals know what qualities and characteristics they want in a romantic partner and consciously evaluate the extent to which the partner fits the bill. They are not rigid; they know that all individuals grow and change over time. Yet they also know that certain core values—honesty, commitment, trustworthiness, integrity, and so forth—are necessary over time. They can imagine worse conditions than being single, such as attempting a long-term romantic relationship without mutual trust and respect.

"Undependence," in cognitive terms, is an acceptance of the premise that relationships, especially romantic relationships, require mutual respect as well as mutual concern. From this basic premise flow all the other aspects of good marriages that therapists usually mention: trust, honesty, commitment, consistency, good communication, and so on. If you respect yourself, and know what you want, then you can respect and love your partner.

It is also advisable to look for the *evidence* to support one's feelings about a romantic partner, especially before allowing oneself to act on such a conclusion. Always looking for evidence before acting on emotional, unexamined conclusions contributes to the development of self-reliance, self-esteem and, as a byproduct, functional relationships.

The Twelve Steps in Perspective

The AA philosophy tries to resolve the fundamental contradiction between self-responsibility and a total surrender to a Higher Power by having a little bit of each. This compromise may sound like a reasonable way to resolve the inevitable clash between science and religion, but it nevertheless remains an incongruity. If AA wants to go the religious route, it must at least provide the methods for helping people have better contact with God, just as other religions have attempted to do for centuries and continue to attempt in the present day. If AA wants to go the science and reason route, then it needs to provide the tools for a rational philosophy of life so that individuals can live happier, more productive lives. But the Twelve Steps approach cannot have it both ways, at least not if it purports to be a coherent and logically consistent philosophy of life.

By rejecting religious faith in favor of reason, I do not mean to imply that the human mind is infallible. I *am* claiming that the potential of the human mind remains vastly underrated. As our culture becomes more suspicious of individualism and rationality, there is a corresponding increase in the flight to irrational psychologies. Increasingly, we look to political leaders, psychotherapists and various spiritual gurus to do for us what we are capable of doing much better for ourselves.

If left unchecked, such a cultural attitude can lead to the decline of civilization as we know it. The decline of reason resulted in the end of the Roman era, followed by the Dark Ages and the bloody, repressive rule of religious dictators; evidence suggests that Western civilization is now headed in a similar direction.[35] In this respect bad therapies, including Twelve Steps therapies based upon illogical dogmas, are helping to accelerate today's widely discussed cultural decline.

I certainly do not wish to suggest that AA should be banned. Advocates of AA have every right to promote their ideas and, despite the flaws in the philosophy, some individuals at least appear to have benefited from participation in a Twelve Step program. But the flaws in the Twelve Steps philosophy are the result of basic logical contradictions, and they need to be exposed as such so the road may be paved for the development of improved treatments for alcoholics and other addicts.

Twelve Steps Therapy and the Addict

It should not be concluded from all of this that any therapist who mentions Twelve Steps, or has some Twelve Steps literature in his office waiting room, should be eliminated from consideration as a good therapist. Many good therapists (including myself) accept the rational aspects of the Twelve Steps for honest and well-intentioned reasons. The essential point remains that the Twelve Steps philosophy consists of contradictory principles. The addict must separate the rational principles from the irrational ones in order to avoid confusion and potential self-harm. Since many therapists of nonaddicted clients also stress the Twelve Steps, all consumers of psychotherapy need to evaluate the steps carefully and critically.

The better Twelve Steps-oriented therapists tend to emphasize the rational, empowering parts of the Twelve Steps rather than surrendering to a Higher Power. Some of these therapists do not even discuss the "Higher Power" aspect, and instead focus on issues such as detachment, devictimizing oneself, and "undependence." Other Twelve Steps therapists, however, might emphasize surrender to a Higher Power as the most important part of psychotherapy.

The addict or otherwise emotionally troubled individual must keep in mind the principles emphasized throughout this book. Any therapy which encourages taking responsibility for one's own life and using rational thought processes rather than merely relying on blind emotions, is likely to be of some help. On the other hand, any therapy which encourages the client to give up self-control and reason to an arbitrarily defined Higher Power quite certainly does damage to the mental health and self-esteem of the client.

The road to psychological helplessness is paved with Higher Powers and spiritual dependence. The road to independence and self-esteem is paved with reliance on one's independent, rational judgment. In the spirit of the latter, allow me to propose a thirteenth step.

Step Thirteen: *Wrote my psychological declaration of independence. I no longer needed to rely on either my feelings or others to make my decisions for me. Came to realize that my own mind, with its capacity to think and reason, was the best method for living and learning. No longer needed therapists, groups—even God—to tell me what to do. Finally lived as an adult man or woman.*

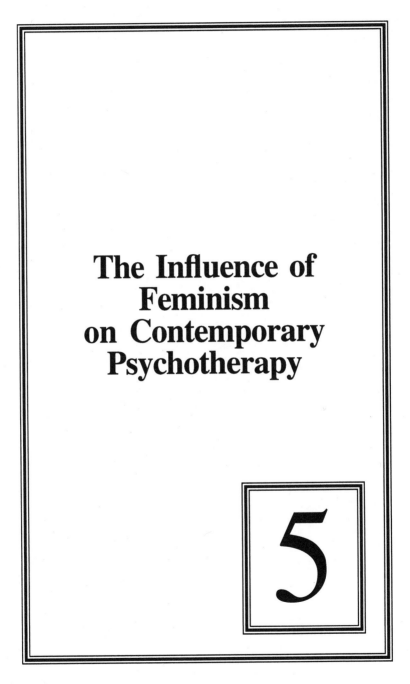

The Influence of Feminism on Contemporary Psychotherapy

5

Because of the various misunderstandings and over-charged emotions surrounding the term "feminism," I will first define the concept clearly. *Rational* feminism refers to the commitment to conscious, objective judgment of women as individuals and *only* as individuals, based upon the facts of reality.

Rational feminists grant no distinctions between men and women except those supported by objective evidence and logic. One can be certain, for example, that men and women possess different reproductive organs and, on the whole, different levels of physical strength. We do not know, however, with any certainty that women and men possess fundamentally different psychological make-ups.

With this rational approach to feminism in mind, we can now properly define the terms "sexism" and "militant feminism."

A sexist viewpoint involves any unwarranted generalization about men-as-a-whole, women-as-a-whole, or both. An unwarranted generalization involves an idea for which insufficient empirical evidence and/or logical validation exists; examples include the notions that women "instinctually" desire to raise children, or that men are wild beasts by nature and only "taming" by women through traditional marriage institutions can save them. "Sexism" refers to an unwarranted generalization about men *or* women, a generalization based upon emotion or superstition rather than actual fact.

Militant feminism, as opposed to rational feminism, represents the dominant form of thinking about gender in today's American culture. Militant feminism differs from rational feminism in that political power and emotional intimidation elevate themselves higher than reason, persuasion and just plain facts.

From the perspective of a rational feminist, militant feminism does almost nothing to correct the traditional understanding of the sexes as members of two logically opposed cultural "universes." Militant feminism instead suggests, and sometimes openly argues, that women are under the power of men whether they know it or not, and that in order to correct this alleged injustice men must be removed from their position of power (by physical force if necessary).

Feminist Marilyn French writes that most men are guilty of violence against women, and that relations between men and women constitute a virtual battlefield.[36] Catherine MacKinnon claims that the essence of femininity in our culture consists of women's accepting and even desiring "male domination."[37] Sandra Lee Bartky agrees, and goes further to suggest that women seize state power to forcibly "reeducate" men.[38]

To further illustrate the militant feminist view that women are, by nature, the victims of men, consider this position on pornography:

> Pornography is an *abuse* of the right to freedom of speech, and the First Amendment was never intended to protect material that condones and promotes violent crimes against any group—be it women, children, Third World people, Jews, old people, etc. The fact

> that the issue of "censorship" is raised so
> readily when women are the victims, in con-
> trast with other groups, suggests that a po-
> litical ploy is being used to confuse and
> intimidate us.[39]

Notice how this statement rests on several emotionally appealing but illogical premises: (1) producers of pornographic material are guilty of "violent crimes"; (2) *all* women are victims of these crimes; and (3) to oppose censorship on principle, even in the case of pornography, amounts to an endorsement of sexism.

These assumptions are easy to refute. First of all, it is illogical to claim that any written or photographic material, however provocative or insensitive, is equivalent to an act of violence or force; after all, do nude models have guns held to their heads or are any women forced to view the pornographic material or pose for it? Clearly, no force is ever involved.

Secondly, even if one concedes the untenable argument that the production and sale of pornographic material itself represents an act of force, it still makes no sense to claim that all women are victims of it; such an assertion blots out the individual identities of millions of women, some of whom live in ignorance of the material, some of whom find it tasteless but not overly offensive, and others who find it offensive but simply resolve not to allow it in their homes, etc.

Finally, without First Amendment protection of pornography the government could interfere in other areas it considers offensive, including the activities and writings of the feminists themselves.

These illogical and mistaken ideas all result from determinism, the same concept that has corrupted psychotherapy and the other social sciences. Determinism ignores or outright rejects the concept of free will, thus allowing one to assert that certain individuals (in this case, women) can be victims even if they are not being forced to do something, such as being forced to read or pose for pornographic publications.

The vague and unsupported references to power and force, so central to all deterministic viewpoints, suggest that women are the helpless byproducts of forces outside of their control and awareness. As one author writes, "Feminist consciousness is consciousness of *victimization* . . . to come to see oneself as a victim" [her emphasis].[40]

Nowhere in the militant feminist literature will one find reference to the idea of free choice or the corresponding idea that women possess the freedom to use their minds and make rational choices just as men do. Instead, the militant feminists focus on the collective victimization of women and the corresponding anger all women supposedly ought to feel toward society as a whole. As one angry feminist put it, "The inequality of women does not arise out of [natural] defect—but rather out of economic, social, political, and legislative default."[41]

Such a statement sets up a false alternative: either women are incompetent by nature, or they are helpless victims of society. It does *not* imply that women, like men, are potentially capable individuals who should therefore be left free and responsible to develop their talents and interests just as men do; instead, the statement implies that government institutions (funded largely through taxing and regulating hated "male" industries) have a moral duty to provide all women with equal status on demand. The logical flaw in this view resides in the fact that if women require equal status on demand, rather than having to earn it, then they must not be capable of genuine achievement in the first place.

While all feminists properly condemn *individual* instances of injustice (such as rape and condescending attitudes toward the abilities of individual women), militant feminists go one step further and insist that such injustices occur because of fundamental psychological differences between men and women.

A typical example of such an assertion is found in the works of popular feminist psychologist Carol Gilligan. Gilligan claims that in childhood boys develop a masculine identity through separating from their mothers while girls develop a feminine identity through becoming close to their mothers. Because of this difference, she concludes, adult men feel that their masculinity is threatened by closeness, while adult women feel that their femininity is threatened by separation.[42] Gilligan's theory, posing as something new and innovative, merely supports and reinforces the old stereotype that men hate intimacy and women dislike independence.

Gilligan's view relies on neo-Freudian theories about the development of the child in early years. Such theories largely rest upon the idea that human relationships are the primary, if not exclusive, arena through which psychological development takes place. This premise contrasts with the cognitive view that the primary agent of psychological development is the thinking human mind; according to cognitive theory, a wealth of assumptions, conclusions and generalizations form the psychological basis for emotional states throughout one's early life, and, subconsciously at least, into the adult years.

The psychodynamic, Freudian view suggests that human personality develops primarily out of early experiences with one's parents, experiences which remain "unconscious" into adulthood and remain difficult, if not impossible, to reverse throughout adult life. The cognitive view, in contrast, suggests that human psychology is the consequence of one's most fundamental conclusions and evaluations and that free will enables the adult man or woman to access

such conclusions, change them as necessary through introspection, and enjoy the corresponding improvements in one's
psychological state.

If one adopts the feminist-psychodynamic view that boys
and girls evolve in fundamentally different ways because of
their early childhood experiences, then the idea that women
are collective victims of male-dominated conventions and
need to find their own "voice" in society becomes easier to
accept. After all, if women cannot help the fact that they
possess psychologically different natures from men, then
insisting that a "woman's" approach to any subject be developed alongside a "man's" approach seems more than
reasonable. Psychologists such as Gilligan conveniently
extend the principle of feminine victimization to the field of
human psychological development, claiming in effect that
women are the victims of psychological theories based upon
"masculine" ideals and "masculine" theories of development. The masculine ideals are tied to objectivity, reason,
and individualism; the feminine ideals are tied to subjectivity, emotionalism and dependence.

Of course, not all feminists adopt the position that individualism and rationality are the domain of men while
caring and attachment are the natural arena of women.
Feminist Betty Friedan, for example, has criticized militant
feminists for rejecting individualism and independence in
favor of government-mandated political coercion.[43] Colette
Dowling, author of *The Cinderella Complex,* in a similar
vein writes that "women have only one real shot at 'liberation,' and that is to emancipate ourselves from within. *It is
the thesis of this book that personal, psychological depen-
dency—the deep wish to be taken care of by others—is the
chief force holding women down today... Like Cinderella,
women today are still waiting for something external to
transform their lives.*" [Emphasis in original][44]

Margaret Talbot, a writer who visited several well-known women's colleges which rely upon militant feminist principles, reacted this way to the intellectual climate of such schools:

> The language of feeling, belief in the bedrock of subjective experience, a kind of *Oprah*-esque confessionalism are given pride of place here and do their part to discourage argument about ideas.[45]

If one approaches the issue of feminism rationally, as Friedan, Dowling and Talbot do in these quotes, one can see that rejecting the militant feminist viewpoint does not mean sexism or bigotry; nor does it mean militant traditionalism. Militant traditionalism refers to the rejection of rationality and objectivity in favor of nostalgia for the past. To the traditionalist, old approaches are good for their own sake, not for any objective reason which stands the test of time.

Militant traditionalism holds that women ought to sacrifice whatever career ambitions they have in favor of having children and "taming" men—all in accordance with their nature as women. Traditionalists generally justify their views by some form of the "Natural Law" argument, the idea that God or some other deterministic force meant for men and women to have certain roles and that such roles must be rigidly maintained even in the midst of spectacular technological and intellectual progression.

Former U.S. Senator Sam Ervin's statement offers a very good illustration of this view. While archaic by current standards, the Senator's ideas about gender are still held by many of today's right-wing religious activists as the ideal:

When He created them, God made physiological and functional differences between
men and women. These differences confer
upon men a greater capacity to perform ar-
duous and hazardous physical tasks. Some
wise people even profess the belief that there
may be psychological differences between
men and women.

To justify their belief, they assert that
women possess an intuitive power to distinguish between wisdom and folly, good and
evil ... From time whereof the memory of
mankind runneth not to the contrary, custom
and law have imposed upon men the primary
responsibility for providing a habitation and
livelihood for their wives and children to
enable their wives to make the habitations
homes, and to furnish nurture, care, and training to their children during their early years.[46]

Ervin's statement provides an excellent example of
nostalgia applied to the subject of gender. He acknowledges, for example, that the notion of fundamental psychological differences between men and women amounts to
mere "belief" or faith; yet in the very same sentence he
refers to individuals holding such a belief as "wise." This
sentimental and naive statement implies that even though
his assertion may stand in opposition to the facts, it nevertheless deserves the respect accorded to hard scientific
knowledge; it is tantamount to saying, "I have no proof for
what I'm claiming, but it feels right so it is therefore wise."

He goes on to confirm the unsupported stereotype that
women rely solely on intuition in order to make discoveries
and even implies that such intuition is actually a higher

form of wisdom than "masculine" wisdom, or rationality! (One wonders if the Senator would have approved of intuition as a method for fighting World War II, or manufacturing cars, or discovering electricity.) Like the militant feminists, he takes it for granted that the most obvious, biological differences between men and women necessarily imply fundamental psychological differences, even though the field of science has not rendered any real evidence to suggest that this is the case.

Remnants of Senator Ervin's irrational sexism undoubtedly remain in our society, even in the "politically correct" university atmospheres of the 1990s. The head of Trinity College, a respected, liberal all girls' school in Washington, D.C., asserts that males are essentially "hierarchical and linear" while females are fundamentally "collaborative and cooperative."[47] If this stereotypical and unwarranted generalization were true, then how do we explain the prevalence of male diplomats and marriage counselors, as well as female physicians, scientists and computer scientists?

In reality, the technological advances in Western civilization have rendered obsolete any previous need for men and women to have a *rigidly* distinguished division of labor, or any distinction based upon physical strength. As Western society has become more rational (via technology, science and free enterprise) in the past several hundred years, the degree of freedom individual women possess for realizing their intellectual potential has grown exponentially. Rationality, logic and science have made the world a better place for women, especially since physical prowess becomes less important in a politically free, scientific culture. Women who today enjoy advancement in the careers of their choice should thank science and economic freedom and not the relentless attacks by feminist intellectuals against masculinity, rationality and the system of free enterprise.

If militant feminists really want to help improve the lives of individual women, they ought to be the strongest proponents of capitalism and rationality. Instead, they often downplay and even belittle the very values of reason and technology that make any form of liberation possible in the first place. Feminist Nora Johnson's view is typical in this regard:

> Feminism is less an I.Q. contest than a system of values for which women are the symbol; strange, outlaw, this system listens to the heart, believes in intuition, is impatient with the rational and the logical, goes for love every time.
>
> It may even be a condition of the soul.[48]

Feminist Madeleine L'Engle has a similar idea:

> My role as a feminist is not to compete with men in their world—that's too easy [!] and ultimately unproductive. My job is to live fully as a woman, enjoying the whole of myself and my place in the universe ... To live in an open and undetermined universe with courage and grace seems to me to epitomize feminine spirituality, and it is the way we are going to have to go if we are to survive as a human race.[49]

Notice how both of these feminists accept as an undisputed axiom that "masculine" and "feminine" natures are fundamentally different, particularly with respect to the issues of rationality and functioning in the real world. Johnson implies that women are intuitive and that intuition is actually superior to reason and logic, at least for women. L'Engle likewise seems to favor rejecting the "masculine" approach to life in favor of the "feminine." While no doubt a great many women feel this way, it seems pointless to consider such viewpoints innovative or even radical.

Although militant feminism and militant traditionalism may often reach different conclusions, their arguments rest upon the same unsubstantiated theories. Militant traditionalists claim that men are by nature more logical and rational than women but at the same time patronize women for their allegedly "intuitive" and emotional natures. Militant feminists likewise accept without question that men are rational by nature and women are emotional by nature; they simply draw a different conclusion: namely, that emotionalism is superior to logic—at least for women. The two approaches are mutually reinforcing and drive men and women further apart, both psychologically and intellectually.

Militant Feminism and the War Against Objectivity and Rationality

A rational philosophy of life, as described in chapter three, helps one understand that no individual need ever be at the mercy of his emotions. Now *this* is liberation—for men as well as for women who struggle with conflicts between thoughts and feelings.

To a great extent contemporary feminist theory presumes that the "masculine" approach to gathering knowledge is objectivity and the "feminine" approach to gathering knowledge is subjectivity. In one study, the feminist authors concluded—from a limited sample of women interviewed on the role of feelings in forming their own value judgments—that women "progress" from an early stage of "received knowledge" (which includes a recognition of objective reality) to a stage of "constructed knowledge" in which all knowledge is seen as subjective.[50]

The study, entitled "Women's Ways of Knowing," leaves the impression that knowledge (for women) can only be based on feelings. By labeling such a transition "progression," the authors clearly imply that the constructed, subjective approach to knowledge is superior to the "received" form of knowledge that included recognition of objective reality.

Because of these inherent differences, according to the authors of the study, men and women should be held to different standards in college education. They view critical reasoning methods, where students are pushed to think logically and defend their ideas, as inherently masculine and inappropriate for women.[51] Imagine the outcry if a group of *male* researchers made such an assertion!

As one critic of this approach says,

> I am not convinced that there *are* any distinctively female "ways of knowing." All *any* human being has to go on, in figuring out how things are, is his or her sensory and introspective experience, and the explanatory theorizing he or she devises to accommodate it; and differences in cognitive style, like differences in handwriting, seem more individual than gender-determined.[52]

Nevertheless, the more militant feminists openly advocate the supremacy of emotions in all decisions at both the individual and political levels. The more moderate feminists imply that some kind of balance between "masculine" objectivity and "feminine" subjectivity needs to be established—a kind of neutered solution to the fundamental psychological differences between men and women.

While there are a wide array of individual authors and viewpoints in the social science literature, both the moderates and the militants share the same mistaken assumption that "male" and "female" ways of thinking are necessarily and logically at odds with one another. As another illustration of this fact, consider the following excerpt from Carol Gilligan:

> As we have listened for centuries to the voices of men and the theories of development that their experience informs, so we have come more recently to notice not only the silence of women but the difficulty in hearing what they say when they speak. Yet in the different voice of women lies the truth of an ethic of care, the tie between relationship and responsibility, and the origins of aggression in the failure of connection. The failure to see *the different reality of women's lives* and to hear the differences in their voices stems in part from the assumption that there is a single mode of social experience and interpretation. By positing instead two different modes, we arrive at a more complex rendition of human experience which sees *the truth of separation and attachment in the lives of women and men and recognizes how these truths are carried by different modes of language and thought.*[53]
> [Italics are mine].

Observe how this passage rests on the subjectivist premise that emotions can be superior to facts. Gilligan claims a "different reality" exists for women. Aside from its implication that men and women are necessarily and logically at odds in the psychological realm, her claim amounts to an outright confession of subjectivism. To Gilligan and other subjectivists, "reality" refers to the state of someone's consciousness rather than facts which exist, objectively, independent of anyone's consciousness. Since men and women appear to reason differently about moral issues, Gilligan maintains, they must be living in two different realities; in other words, men and women are fundamentally and hopelessly different.

Gilligan's thesis, quoted above, represents the climax of a study in which she attempts to make the case that women adopt an "ethic of care" while men adopt an "ethic of justice." Gilligan's study, a highly influential one among psychologists and psychotherapists since the 1980s, sets up a viciously false alternative: not only between "male" and "female" approaches to morality but also between the attributes of "care" and "justice."

Such a false alternative implies that an individual cannot be *both* caring and just. Caring, in this context, presumably means an emphasis on compassion and feelings, while justice presumably refers to an emphasis on objectivity and observation of the facts (as in a courtroom or scientific laboratory). In other words, men by nature prefer facts and women by nature prefer feelings. Gilligan, while attempting to arrive at "a more complex rendition of human experience," instead merely restates the so-called wisdom of the ages by reinforcing the unsubstantiated, sexist view that women are feelers and men are thinkers.

Gilligan's error betrays a still deeper misunderstanding about the true definition of objectivity and rationality. Most individuals think of rationality as being necessarily cold, uncaring and indifferent to feelings. "He's so *rational*," is more often meant as an insult than a compliment, especially when uttered by feminist-traditionalists who subscribe to the view that men and women inhabit different cultural universes. Yet, as already pointed out in chapter three, true rationality does not lead to coldness or repression of feelings, nor are repression and denial indicative of a healthy psychological state.

Militant feminists and like-minded intellectuals have perpetuated the idea that rationality/productivity and "social welfare" are mutually exclusive. Consider the example of capitalistic "exploitation," usually condemned as evil for its focus on technology at the expense of humanity. Men and women benefit daily, in reality, from the fact that oil fields have been exploited, and that other natural resources have been exploited to provide the countless comforts and life-sustaining technologies of modern civilization. Rationality does not represent all that is evil in human beings; on the contrary, it represents all that saves human beings from evil and destruction, both from within and without.

Despite these facts militant feminism has delivered near-fatal blows to the reputation of rationality in recent decades. First, feminism incorrectly accepts the premise of the traditionalists that women are inherently irrational or, at best, less rational by nature than are men. Embittered by this alleged fact, feminists then (in varying degrees) turn on rationality by claiming, in effect, that "if women can't be rational, then being rational is evil." Militant feminism, like traditionalism, takes it for granted that women are basically incapable of being rational—and, instead of confining women to the kitchen and to sewing circles, have decided instead to pursue a course of destroying everything associated (accurately or not) with the notion of masculinity.

Because rationality and masculinity are so intimately (and inaccurately) associated, it should come as no surprise when militant feminists viciously attack the social mechanisms which rationality most requires: the free market system, the political principle of absolute freedom upon which the market depends, and the once admired/now despised psychological traits of independence, self-esteem and self-reliance upon which freedom depends. If men are inherently rational, and if women are inherently intuitive and subjectivist, then it makes sense to attack the free market system. After all, the free market system places responsibility on the individual man or woman for earning his or her own living without handouts or enforced "charity" from others. The feminist-socialists who believe that women are innately helpless victims of forces beyond their control are at least logically consistent in supporting some form of government control. As one such feminist writes,

> The nature of women's oppression is unique; women are oppressed as women, regardless of class or race; some women have access to significant wealth, but that wealth does not signify power; women are to be found everywhere, but own or control no appreciable territory; women live with those who oppress them, sleep with them, have their children— we are tangled, hopelessly it seems, in the gut of the machinery and way of life which is ruinous to us.[54]

If femininity and the free market system of property rights are fundamentally incompatible, as this quotation clearly implies they are, then it makes total sense to condemn such a system as sexist.

Yet, if women have choices and are capable of practicing a rational philosophy of life, then just the opposite is true: women, because of certain inaccurate ideas and unfair laws in the past, now require freedom perhaps *more* desperately than men if they can expect to live happy, productive, and self-sustaining lives. Only through challenging the idea that women are inherently irrational, therefore, will more women see that free market individualism serves their interest far better than any other social system.

The appropriate alternative to the irrational versions of both feminism and traditionalism is, once again, the rational approach to life. The rational approach sets for both men and women the goal of establishing psychological harmony between one's emotions and one's thoughts through the process of introspection. Of course human beings are capable of evil, ugly things, such as rape or blindly evasive racism or sexism. But these evils can only be conquered by cold, rational logic, and not by the very forms of evasion and emotionalism which gave rise to such ideologies in the first place.

A rational approach to the masculine/feminine psychology issue would help end pointless political and psychological squabbles over what "men" want and what "women" want. Even if objective psychological differences between men and women are ultimately shown to exist, such discoveries will not undermine the following principle: rationality serves the long-term individual interest of both men and women; the irrational clinging to unsubstantiated theories, old or "new," creates nothing except long-term despair, disillusionment and cynicism.

Until enough people recognize and accept that both men *and* women think *and* feel, there will be no liberation for anyone. Bad therapy based upon militant feminism and "women's ways of knowing" only makes matters worse. As Margaret Talbot writes, "Spreading the message that traits like cooperativeness and competitiveness are gender-coded, pink and blue, is risky business. It threatens to revive old stereotypes of women as gentle, intuitive caretakers and men as tough-minded aggressors."[55]

Militant Feminism and Bad Therapy

It is important to understand two points about militant feminism and psychotherapy. First, a therapist may appear to be a reasonable individual and still share the erroneous premises of the militant feminist ideology. Second, the basic theories of militant feminism have become so ingrained in our cultural institutions—especially in the humanities departments of most major universities—that only the most individualistic students of psychology will ever dare question them.

Given these two points, it should not surprise anyone that so many therapists operate on the premises of militant feminism, often without fully realizing it. The psychotherapy profession often attracts amiable, congenial individuals who do not want to upset the status quo. And make no mistake about it: watered-down militant feminism embodies the status quo of today's social science disciplines and, increasingly, society-at-large. The world has rarely, if ever, been witness to a more philosophically entrenched establishment than today's "politically correct" ideologies to which social scientists are increasingly exposed in their university training.[56] The client should understand the nature of these ideas so that she can (1) judge for herself their validity or lack thereof, and (2) assess to what extent, if any, her particular therapist relies upon them when providing guidance.

The basic assumptions underlying militant feminism (insofar as it affects psychotherapy) are as follows:

The deterministic view. According to this view, both men and women are the product of inescapable social conditioning.

In reality, no free individual, male or female, is the product of inescapable social conditioning. Children made to feel like worthless "nobodies" can, and often do, grow up to accomplish great things. Other children who receive everything from their parents can, and often do, fail miserably in life. The overwhelming majority of children in urban ghettos do *not* grow up to be criminals. Women accomplished great things in science and business long before the women's movement of the 1970s. Clearly social learning, while a relevant factor, is not the determining factor in the development of individual health and self-esteem.

Good therapy does not fall into the trap of any form of determinism, including the militant feminist variety. A good therapist assumes that individuals have choices and that therapy should enhance, rather than destroy, the individual's confidence in making good choices for himself or herself. The client must evaluate her therapy carefully, asking herself the following questions: "Am I being taught to set goals (in career or elsewhere), and learning to better cope with my emotions? Or am I losing sight of these goals due to an over-emphasis on the differences between men and women in society and how this can be expected to inhibit me? Is therapy giving me an idea of how to be rational and successful—or simply how to be *angry?*" The client should not answer these questions quickly, but instead keep them in mind as therapy progresses.

The "different voice" view. The "different voice" view refers to the idea, discussed earlier in this chapter, that men and women are fundamentally different psychologically. Proponents of this theory generally take it for granted that men are essentially logical and women are essentially intuitive; they merely criticize what they see as a negative bias against intuition in favor of rationality.

Feminist Carol Gilligan, for instance, does not criticize existing theory and research for stereotyping women as innately "intuitive" or "instinctive"; instead, she accepts this premise and simply criticizes prior researchers for not granting intuition and instinct equal status with rationality.[57]

This claim is reasonable and justified *if* one accepts that women are by nature intuitive and instinctive. If women cannot help their emotionalist nature, after all, then it certainly is not fair to penalize them by trying to fit them into a rational, "male" theory of moral or psychological development.

Undeniably, both biological and social differences between men and women do exist. Children, of course, are influenced by the ideas their elders teach about the sexes. If parents teach their daughters that it is unnatural for women to become scientists or astronauts, for example, their daughters may accept this assertion uncritically. But the adult woman can overcome such injustices through independent thinking and through *reason*—especially if rationality is valued (and not mocked as anti-female) by the thinkers and teachers who influence her throughout adolescence and young adulthood.

Does the "different voice" idea have consequences for psychotherapy clients? Absolutely; most therapists, in my experience, implicitly accept the idea that men and women are psychologically different. This leads them to grant equal or, in some cases, even superior status to unexamined emotions as opposed to careful reasoning. Consider the following concrete examples.

> The marriage counselor who asks the husband to equate his wife's feelings with facts, without expecting the wife to provide the reasons and justifications for why her emotions are true;

> The psychotherapist who encourages his female client to leave her husband for no other reason than "I don't feel that I'm in love with him anymore," without first helping the client clarify her definition of love and determining for what reasons she thinks her current relationship does not and cannot fit into those criteria;

> The group therapist who tells her client that
> not only does she have a right to express her
> feelings in the group, but that she has a cor-
> responding right to have her feelings accepted
> as valid.

Therapists with a feminist orientation will often encourage their female clients (individually or in all-female groups) simply to "go with their feelings" and not pay any heed to the request of others (especially their husbands) that they provide some logical basis for their feelings. While presumably such therapists only want to make their clients more independent, they actually encourage them to be more *dependent.* The only way to independence and self-esteem is through the adoption of a rational philosophy of life. A rational philosophy of life requires a recognition that feelings do not always conform to objective facts and that a process of rational introspection must be utilized to distinguish between perception and reality.

If we are to create a non-sexist world where men and women respect each other as unique individuals, then both men *and* women must rely on a rational philosophy of life in order to survive and flourish. The militant feminist psychotherapist cuts off this possibility by treating women as helpless, embittered victims and dismissing reason as if it were unhealthy, sexist and outdated.

So long as the "different voice" premise remains unchallenged in the academic culture where psychotherapists are trained, militant feminism will continue to exercise an influence on the therapy process. Psychotherapy clients should therefore remember that good therapy poses neither "masculinity" nor "femininity" as the ideal. Good therapy is nonsexist. It encourages *both* men and women to identify and be aware of their feelings yet at the same time think about their feelings using logical standards.

Men, as a whole, have generally been trained to repress and ignore feelings; women, as a whole, have generally been taught to overemphasize feelings. Neither has been taught how to introspect and actually reason with his or her feelings. In the area of psychological health, therefore, both men and women have been victimized by wrong ideas and have a long road still to travel. A wise and understanding therapist sees beneath the cynical veneer of today's "war between the sexes" and understands that men *and* women need to learn how to handle their feelings more appropriately.

The victim view. According to the victim view, all women are victims of society's unfair attitudes. As one feminist put it,

> In a consciousness raising group, women discuss their own feelings and experiences. In discussing how similar these are from woman to woman, women discover the political nature of their problems. The individual woman learns that she is not a misfit, a kook, or sick but rather that society is sick.[58]

Generally left out of this view is a coherent definition of society. What is society, anyway? One rational definition refers to "a given number of individuals who comprise a geographic area or social group." Yet the concept "society" is often used by militant feminists to mean some kind of imaginary masculine monster whose destruction would result in a utopia for all.

In reality, no individual—male or female—can be a victim of society. One *can* be a victim of a particular person or a group of persons (the examples of theft, fraud, rape, blackmail or murder come to mind). But unless one actually experiences victimization by every single individual (or most individuals) in the country at the same time, it makes no sense to speak of victimization by "society."

Nor can one truly be a victim of "society's attitudes," despite what many feminist-oriented therapists claim. Attitudes refer to the ideas or feelings of certain individuals. "Society's attitudes" presumably refer to the ideas and feelings of a majority of individuals in a particular social group. Even if a woman holds a different view from every other person on the planet, nobody can force her to think in a certain way. If she is not independent enough to think for herself, it is still not appropriate to call her a victim. Independent thinking, while never easy, can be encouraged by teaching young boys and girls to use their minds and logical reasoning abilities.

Militant feminist intellectuals and psychotherapists operate on the assumption that women are victims of certain inaccurate or unproven stereotypes. Instead of merely attempting to correct invalid stereotypes through logical persuasion, however, they adopt a stance of revenge-seeking. According to the revenge-seeking viewpoint, *all* women represent victims and *all* men represent aggressors. In any particular situation, whether it be the Clarence Thomas nomination to the Supreme Court or a couple in a marriage counseling office, the usual standards of objectivity and proof are replaced with emotional agendas. In a divorce, for example, angry feminist judges view the husband as the aggressor and the wife as the victim—and they often divide both property and children accordingly. Feminist therapists use their clout as "experts" to reinforce this false idea throughout the court system. I see evidence of this trend in my practice.

Therapists who encourage the victim view do their clients a disservice. We know from research studies that an exaggerated feeling of powerlessness and helplessness lies at the root of depression and many other mental health problems.[59] Victim-oriented therapists simply reinforce their client's feelings of powerlessness by blaming everything on society. Through reinforcing the very distorted thought processes they ought to be challenging, victim-oriented therapists can do irreparable harm to their clients.

One cannot carry the feminist "victim" notion to its logical conclusion without frightening consequences for everyone. At the same time, many feminists—with the full endorsement of many therapists—seek to do precisely this. In 1988, for example, a California judge set aside a jury conviction of murder in the case of a "24-year-old woman who had argued that she was suffering from 'baby blues' [or postpartum depression] when she ran her automobile over her infant son and then left the body in a trash can."[60]

Taken to its only possible conclusion, the feminist "victim" view results in such court decisions. And given the all-encompassing influence of feminist ideas on today's psychiatric profession and the fact that courts rely heavily on the so-called "authority" of psychiatric testimony in such cases, we can probably expect many more such decisions in the future. The victim view, so eloquently demonstrated by this case, involves the characterization of a woman as so helpless and so determined by her emotions that she cannot even be expected to refrain from running her baby over with an automobile. Women, such decisions often imply, are not responsible for their actions; and paternalistic male judges, politicians and psychotherapists fall for it. This is what feminism defines as "liberation" for women?

In the short-run, victimization status may bring a false sense of self-esteem and security to an emotionally troubled person. We live, after all, in the Age of Victimization: one is elevated to the status of a celebrity simply for having been sexually or otherwise abused as a child. In the long-run, though, nothing (not even decades of psychotherapy) can replace a conviction that one has the free will to act and achieve successfully in life. This conviction develops through the active use of one's mind and one's actual efforts to achieve goals. A woman always encouraged to go with her feelings and to ignore rationality can still learn how to think better. A man always encouraged to ignore his feelings at any price can also learn to become a healthier, integrated person. Most men *and* women need to learn how to introspect and become more fully rational, integrated individuals. Women do not hold a monopoly on growing up with bad ideas.

Feminist psychotherapists may sincerely want to help their clients. Or they may want to indoctrinate them with ideas which, repackaged in intellectual sounding terms, are simply variations on the same old themes. Either way, victim-oriented feminist psychotherapy is psychologically unhealthy. It is unhealthy to see oneself as a helpless creature determined by "society." Women, especially, cannot afford to adopt such a view in a world where they are increasingly responsible for supporting themselves financially and psychologically.

The separatist view. According to this view, men and women are thought to inhabit separate cultural universes. Such an idea has been around for a long time. In earlier eras, women sat in their sewing circles and men on their bar stools and each discussed the hopeless differences between the two genders. Today, feminist therapists and their female clients complain about how "insensitive" men are while their husbands beat on drums and perform tribal rituals at a men's "therapy" group down the street. At least the sewing circles and bar stools of yesteryear did not cost $100 per hour!

M. Carey Thomas, the founder of Bryn Mawr College in 1885, said that her overriding aim in establishing an all-female college was "to show that girls can learn, can reason, can compete with men in the grand fields of literature and science and conjecture."[61] According to historians,

Thomas neither recognized nor endorsed the notion of a special feminine nature. Today's proponents of different voices and women's ways of knowing could learn from an innovative thinker such as Thomas.

The separatist vision relies, ultimately, on the false idea that men and women live in different "realities." Nothing can change the fact that there is only *one* reality, and both men and women have to live in it. As long as militant feminist therapists continue insisting that raw feeling and ill-defined "caring" are superior to reason and logic, all the while implying that feeling and caring are naturally feminine traits, they only dig themselves deeper and deeper into a hole they will repeatedly deny exists.

The strength in numbers view. Proponents of militant feminism claim they only want to educate society about mistaken sexist ideas. While on the surface a seemingly reasonable goal, such feminists really want the freedom to spread their ideas as "scientific" without having to accept responsibility for submitting all of these ideas to a rigorous scientific process. They want to establish as scientific *fact,* for example, that "attitudes" and "society" victimize women, despite the lack of evidence for such claims. They want others to accept as scientific *fact,* rather than opinion, that men and women are products of inescapable social conditioning, despite insufficient evidence to warrant such a conclusion. In the heat of debate, they may even brand as "sexist" and "reactionary" anyone who dares introduce the possibility that their conclusions are incorrect.

Because psychotherapy remains a young science, feminist therapists (and all bad therapists) can often get away with unfair and unchallenged standards. Since the scientific investigation of gender is only in its infancy, pseudo-experts can easily make false claims to the truth when their real motive involves advancing irrational agendas. Following this course of action, many feminist therapists use the respect granted to them by their innocent and uneducated victims to assert their unfounded opinions as scientific facts.

Women who want and need psychological help but are turned off by the victimization approach ought to consider rationality and independence as alternatives. For inspiration they might read about individual examples of women who succeed on their own. They might consider the case of Marie Curie, the Polish scientist who played an instrumental role in the discovery of radioactivity; or Maria Mitchell, the first female astronomer; or nineteenth-century businesswoman Madame C. J. Walker, the first black millionaire; or Lucy Hobbes, the first female dentist; or Maggie Lena Walker, the first female bank president; or Rita Levi-Montalcini, winner of the 1986 Nobel Prize for Physiology/Medicine.[62] Few of these women, or any individual of great accomplishment, likely subscribed to a victimization view.

In therapy, my female clients often discover that the men in their lives, whatever their shortcomings, can also be quite vulnerable. Despite conventional wisdom, most men do not seek to dominate and control their wives. Many men feel confused and, like many women, threatened by the perceived loss of intimacy and closeness when communication breaks down.

My everyday clinical experience, contrary to the feminist doctrines I was taught in graduate school, suggests that most men *want* to be good fathers, even though they are often unsure how to proceed. While some men are stubborn and irrational, fighting irrationality with militant feminism is not the answer.

No client should let a therapist decide whether or not she should stay in a marriage. (A good therapist, by the way, will not want to make this decision for anyone.) Clients and therapists should question the assumption of the militant feminist movement that the universe is a conflict-ridden place where men and women are necessarily and forever at odds with one another. Each case of "man" and "woman" merits individual consideration before making hasty generalizations.

Clients need to remember too that most therapists serve as guardians of the intellectual status quo, which right now happens to consist of watered-down militant feminism. Although reasonable people have dismissed the anti-male philosophies of the 1960s and 1970s, these ideas still represent the foundation for many of today's psychotherapies and self-help books. A bad therapist will base his or her evaluations and recommendations on the false assumptions discussed in this chapter. This fact places added responsibility on the client for evaluating the therapist's philosophy about the nature of women and men.

Feminist Therapy in Action

Battered women's groups. Many—but not necessarily all—battered women's groups adopt the feminist victim view wholeheartedly. Perhaps this fact is understandable, to a point, given that many women who attend such groups are genuine victims. Perhaps through honest ignorance or inexperience they entered a relationship with a man who turned out to be physically abusive. Now they face both psychological and financial dilemmas about what to do next. In theory, battered women's groups offer a unique opportunity to provide such women with some of the tools for developing a rational philosophy of life. Groups using a rational approach could be enormously empowering and liberating for such women.

Unfortunately, many of these groups pursue the militant feminist route instead of the empowerment route. Either directly or indirectly, they encourage victimized women to adopt the view that they must fight "male oppression" rather than the wrong ideas which led them to pursue or maintain such relationships in the first place. Some therapists suggest that merely to *hint* at some responsibility on the part of the abuse victim amounts to "blaming the victim" and must not even be considered. While therapists may well blame the victim at times, and such errors undoubtedly occurred a great deal before physical and sexual abuse was discussed openly, it makes no sense to conclude that battered women are incapable of making any rational choices.

The problem of battered wives should not be transformed from a social problem into a "disease," as is so popular today. "Battered spouse syndrome" does not refer to a disease, although it is probably only a matter of time before the American Psychiatric Association labels it as one.

Nor does the real cure of battered women consist of therapies based upon the emasculation of men. Violent and abusive men are not really masculine. Abusive, irrational men are merely children in men's bodies, pathetic and emotionally retarded specimens of masculinity.

Battered women must learn to let go of mistaken assumptions such as, (1) "all men are brutes, so why bother leaving him? I won't do any better," or (2) "I can make him better if only I love him hard enough. Love will conquer all." Until a woman sees that such deeply held assumptions are mistaken, it is difficult to imagine why she would leave the abusive environment. Therapists, therefore, need to be careful not to encourage the idea that most men are jerks; if a battered wife already thinks that most men are jerks, then it is easier for her to rationalize that she might as well stay with her current husband since it's better than being alone.

Another trend I have observed over ten years of practice is the failure of many therapists to involve the abusers (or husbands) in the treatment process. Although it is very difficult to convince abusive men to become involved in therapy, many therapists do not try hard enough. Such a trend overlooks several important facts: (1) both wife and husband are psychologically invested in the marital relationship by virtue of the time spent in it, and may possess at least some reasonable motives for continuing under new rules; (2) sometimes wives initiate the process of physical violence, and do not merely act out of self-defense; (3) while some violent men will probably never change, some are sincerely awakened by the onset of legal intervention and the threat of losing their children, and deserve a fair hearing from a good therapist. The word "therapy" means "change"—why does "change" *necessarily* mean the break-up of a marriage, especially when children are involved, as opposed to radical changes in the way the couple communicates (i.e., non-violently)? Chances are that each spouse will have to learn new methods of communicating anyway, with new spouses. Why the rush to break up marriages and families indiscriminately?

Battered-spouse therapy, furthermore, often falls into the advice-giving trap. The advice-oriented therapist in the battered spouse treatment center is typically pushy and bossy. She probably means well. She probably has strong feelings about helping women who are abused and have no place to turn. But in her zeal she may forget that the central purpose of therapy consists in helping her client become more self-reliant. The advice-oriented therapist is very opinionated. Good therapists do express their opinions to clients, but they also need to remember that the client must learn to make better decisions with her own independent, rational judgment.

Some battered-spouse therapists overemphasize feelings. They encourage the client to express her feelings of anger and hatred toward her husband, feelings which she may have been too scared to express before. But after the initial feeling of support and relief brought about by such a process, the client may start to wonder what the point of it all is. "Be angry, be angry," is a consistent and initially helpful message to an individual who used to not let herself be angry about anything. But how can she move on with her life by simply remaining angry? And how is she to change her behavior in the future simply by feeling the old feelings over and over again? A feeling-centered therapist, since he does not recognize or acknowledge the difference between thoughts and feelings, cannot help the client determine her mistaken assumptions so that she can better cope in the future.

Other bad therapists ignore the role that the victim's behavior might have played in maintaining the abuse. This does not mean that the victim's husband was justified in hitting her, and this fact must be made explicitly clear; the victim has to remember that violent behavior is never appropriate except in self-defense. At the same time, a good therapist will also help the client look beyond the obvious facts that her husband behaved brutally. A good therapist encourages the victim to understand what led her to stay quiet for as long as she did. What led her to feel guilty when there was no reason to feel guilty? What led her to think that love would conquer everything? Has she now been convinced that love is not enough—that love also requires a non-violent commitment between two individuals? Is it really better to be with someone abusive than to be alone? Are there not worse things than being alone?

Advocacy-oriented therapists in battered spouse facilities sometimes have unspoken personal agendas. Perhaps they want to see as many men as possible put in jail or stripped of their property. Perhaps they are concerned about what they call "social justice." Perhaps they want to take over for the victim altogether. If so, the victim has really exchanged one form of dependence—on a violent, emotionally immature husband—for another form—on an angry therapist who likes to take over for people.

The client should ask herself if the therapist is really helping her or simply trying to prove some kind of point. If there exists actual evidence that the therapist is helping the client become more independent and self-reliant, the client ought to feel pleased. But if anger itself has become the central focus of therapy, then therapy probably does little for the victim over the long-run.

Past-centered therapists encourage the victim to focus almost exclusively on family background issues. To a certain extent this focus on the past is helpful. The victim might learn, for example, how her father's violent nature influenced her choice of a husband who was also violent. But the past-centered therapy stops here. It does not go much beyond the recognition that childhood influences are important. It is not suggested that mistaken conclusions about the nature of men or intimacy may have been formed in childhood, and that such conclusions can be questioned and changed as an adult.

Women's support groups or "women's issues" therapy groups. Some of these groups are highly productive. They can help women learn, as individuals, to pursue their goals and provide a context in which women may share strategies for achieving them. They can provide a sense of emotional support which they may not have received elsewhere. The therapist or group leader does everything possible to encourage such support, and takes responsibility for not allowing the group to degenerate into a complaining, self-pitying hostility-fest directed primarily against men and society.

Unfortunately, not all such groups operate this way. Militant feminist support groups, as already pointed out, may exist to advance the political or psychological agenda of the group therapist. Even when not politically oriented, such groups often utilize the "different voice" notion of "masculine" and "feminine" approaches to thinking and members fume over why men do not simply adopt the "feminine" approach so that everything could be simpler. The self-herding into therapy groups based upon "sisterhood" or "support," furthermore, runs the psychological risk of de-individualizing women. Advocates of feminism during the climate of change in the 1960s and early 1970s, when these groups first began to form, missed out on an historic opportunity. Instead of emphasizing the individualistic idea that women, as well as men, can unleash their potential through self-reliance and rationality, many feminists rebelled against individualism as both masculine and inhuman.

Only a fresh approach to psychology, grounded in a rational philosophy of life, can hope to advance the interests of both men and women in the future. Once the militant feminist ideology is unmasked for the raw traditionalism which it truly is—the idea that women are basically helpless, emotionalist victims and men are uncaring, insensitive monsters—it will be possible for rational feminist intellectuals and therapists to make a worthwhile contribution to the social sciences.

Psychodynamic/"insight" therapy. Although militant feminists generally accuse Sigmund Freud's psychodynamic theories of sexism, feminist therapists often apply Freud's techniques in their own treatments.

Feminism and Freud, who developed the preposterous theory that women envy men for their penises, might seem like strange bedfellows at first glance; but the match is actually a pretty logical one. Both Freudian therapy and militant feminist therapy epitomize *determinism:* the view, once again, that adults are largely or exclusively the byproduct of external forces outside of their control.

The Freudian sees humans as the product of childhood influences; the militant feminist sees humans as the product of gender and social factors. Thus, a feminist therapist can probably find some evidence of male dominance and oppression in the childhood of nearly any female client. Absent fathers represent typical, uncaring males who damage a girl's self-esteem by refusing to love her. Fathers who give their daughters too much attention must be sexual molesters. The increased attention on therapists who hastily conclude that clients were molested as children[63] stems from a potent mixture of Freudianism and feminism. Freudianism-feminist therapists simply blend the idea that women are natural victims with the view that all children want to sleep with their opposite-sex parent at the age of four.

Potential clients must understand that both Freudian and feminist therapists have a *vested interest* in their deterministic theories. If individuals are the helpless byproducts of their childhoods and/or centuries of male oppression, then benevolent authority figures must exist to help such creatures through life. Militant feminist and Freudian therapists undoubtedly see themselves as ideal candidates for this task.

Freudian and feminist therapies inevitably become authoritarian by the very nature of their theories. Human beings, according to their theories, are poor, helpless creatures. All helpless creatures need extensive supervision and control. One form of such supervision involves a psychotherapeutic process in which the therapist allegedly has inherently superior wisdom to the client; not simply more knowledge—but *intrinsically* superior ability.

Left unanswered, of course, is what should be an obvious question: if *all* human beings are helpless, then what makes these therapists (or other authorities) equipped to help the helpless? As depraved human beings, are they not helpless themselves? If not, then what criteria can prove them superior to their inferior clients?

Conclusion

The prospective therapy client needs to be aware of the militant feminist ideas guiding the practice of contemporary psychotherapy. The prospective client also needs to be prepared to evaluate these ideas and understand the hidden implications within them.

The cognitive approach to therapy relies upon the assumption that men and women are equally capable of learning to introspect and reason with their emotions. Its practitioners do not generally become sidetracked by concerns about victimization, social attitudes, penis envy, and women's ways of knowing.

Those who would claim that cognitive therapy is male-oriented or biased against women are merely revealing their own latent sexism; in order to make such a criticism, one must first possess the idea that women are incapable of being rational and in control of their emotional states. Given the success many of my female clients have enjoyed in cognitive therapy, I am convinced that nothing could be further from the truth.

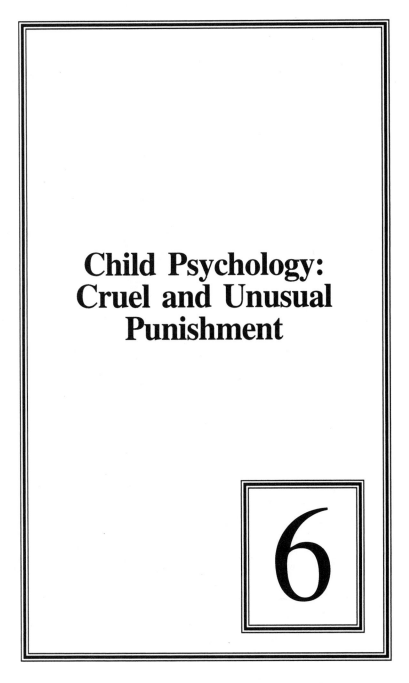

Child Psychology:
Cruel and Unusual
Punishment

6

T he unmotivated child or adolescent is generally not a good candidate for exclusively one-on-one psychotherapy.

There are many reasons for this fact. First of all, if the child or teen has not been listening to or talking with his parents, he is unlikely to talk to a therapist whom his parents have hired to make him talk. And even if for some reason the child does open up honestly and develops a good relationship with the therapist—as most parents initially fantasize that he will—it still does little of lasting consequence to repair the family tensions which drove the parents to seek help in the first place. At best, it can serve as a prelude to family therapy, in which the grievances of each family member become the focus of attention.

In some cases, particularly with angry or obnoxious adolescents, one-on-one therapy can actually create new problems. The manipulative child or adolescent will seize any opportunity to "con" a naive therapist into accepting his point of view while he leaves out important details that might lead the therapist to a different conclusion.

Consider the case of the seventeen-year-old girl who made a fairly convincing argument that her parents were callous and insensitive. Despite the fact that she obtained good grades and did all of her chores, they would not even listen to her requests to attend a good college and have use of a family car. When the therapist met with the parents, however, he discovered that their daughter had also been fired from several jobs for stealing and had been experimenting with marijuana and cocaine. Their daughter had not overtly lied to the therapist, but she had left out important information which would have led him to a significantly different conclusion. A naive, strictly one-on-one adolescent therapist would have developed an alliance with this highly manipulative young woman without knowing all the facts.

Another difficulty with one-on-one therapy involves its encouragement of the usually mistaken idea that the child is at fault for all of the family's problems. While problem children sometimes *do* represent the cause of the family's predicament, a good therapist must also consider many other potential factors. Is the parents' marriage troubled? If so, children will often misbehave as a method of distracting attention away from the problems in the marriage.[64] Do the parents have inaccurate thinking habits which have rubbed off on the child? Sometimes parents are irrational or manipulative, and viewed in the larger context of the family environment, the child's psychological symptoms make a lot of sense. Or do family members simply not know how to communicate with one another? Many families resort to shouting and even physical violence as a means of venting frustrations which would be better handled rationally.

I have interviewed many adults who still express hurt and bitterness over having been dragged to an individual therapist as a child with no explanation on the part of either parents or therapist as to why they were there. Such action sends an early message to a child that forces other than justice and reason are governing her life, and as an adult the child may develop an irrational mistrust of helping professionals and other authorities.

No good therapist, in my opinion, would ever want to see a child individually without (a) providing a good, logical reason for doing so, and (b) at least meeting or speaking with other household members to understand more thoroughly the context in which the child's behavioral or emotional problems occur. Providing *strictly* individual therapy for the child is a neutral form of mental health treatment at best and at its worst can seriously damage a child's self-esteem and sense of justice.

In my practice I have discovered that many parents simply want a baby-sitting service; without even admitting this motive to themselves, they hire therapists to do the job of parenting for them. Indeed, the high prices therapists charge can be rationalized to assuage the guilt such parents feel for what they are doing: "If the therapy costs this much, it must be something good for my child."

Individual child therapy enables parents to become less engaged with their children than they should be. In such cases, too, therapy becomes part of the problem rather than part of the solution. The important thing to realize is that therapy is not a baby-sitting service. A *good* therapist will never allow the process to be treated as such. Parents seriously concerned about their child's emotional or behavioral symptoms need to cooperate with and participate in their child's mental health treatment. When a parent feels helpless, the last thing she needs is a therapist to take over, however tempting this may seem.

Is Individual Therapy
Ever Appropriate for Children?

Individual child therapy may be appropriate, or even necessary, under one or more of the following conditions:

1. The child is sincerely motivated to seek help on his own. Such motivation generally does not occur before the early twenties. In unusual cases, teenagers may exhibit genuine motivation for therapy. One way to test the teenager's sincerity is to allow him to pay for therapy. Most of today's managed-care insurance plans have small co-payments, making it affordable for the adolescent who has a job or an allowance. Even if it is impossible for him to afford therapy on his own, the teenager should still be expected to pay the parents back in some way—through extra work around the house or baby-sitting younger siblings, for example.

I do not recommend individual therapy for any teenager unless he or she is functioning reasonably well in school and is both accepting and handling responsibility for age-appropriate tasks such as household chores, and so on. An adolescent can legitimately pursue individual sessions for such issues as career planning, sexuality, peer issues, or stress.

2. Individual child therapy as part of family therapy. In such cases the therapist retains use of her professional judgment as to when, if ever, to violate confidentiality between herself and the child. The child cannot place the therapist in an ethical dilemma by telling her that she uses drugs, for example, and then insisting this fact not be revealed to the parent, citing state laws on client-therapist confidentiality. The therapist reserves the right to reveal facts given to her by the child, but only under unusual circumstances and with adequate warning, when possible, to the child or teen.

A variation of this approach would involve two different therapists who have obtained written consent from all parties to allow for unrestricted communication between them, as they see fit.

3. Assessment of situations in which the individual rights of a child are at stake. Suspected physical and/or sexual abuse represent the most obvious examples under this category. Nevertheless, a good therapist uses extreme caution in dealing with such highly-charged emotional issues. She recognizes how crucial it is to remain objective, interested only in gathering facts and evidence, and not letting any preconceived notions interfere with the process. A good therapist understands and appreciates that lives can be needlessly destroyed if careful evaluations are not made in such serious matters. It is important in such cases to rely on therapists with a reputation for objectivity and a great deal of experience in dealing with these kinds of issues. Second opinions are also highly recommended.

Good Family Therapy versus Bad Family Therapy

The Permissive Therapist

Bad family therapists are permissive at heart. Permissive refers to the idea that no rational criteria exist for judging something as "good" or "bad," "right" or "wrong"; instead, they exploit the notion that individuals each have their own particular feelings which must be accepted *uncritically* by everyone else.

Permissiveness rejects (or ignores) the idea that feelings are simply automatic versions of subconscious thoughts and premises. It leads to the moral and social relativism so characteristic of modern society: what's right for you and what's right for me are not necessarily the same thing. Since individuals *feel* differently, there must be many different realities.

It is of course true that what's right for you and what's right for me might indeed involve different things. Perhaps you can be a basketball player and I can be a physics teacher. Perhaps I like chocolate ice cream and you prefer strawberry. But permissive therapists are not simply talking about choices and preferences: they are rejecting (or ignoring) the wider distinction between objectively known truths and mere feelings. Once they eliminate this distinction, how can a parent judge when his children are behaving reasonably and when they are not? How can a child learn any rational concept of "right" or "wrong?"

The permissive family therapist assumes that the family must literally consist of a "democracy." Instead of ruling themselves by vote, however, such families actually rule by range-of-the-moment feelings or whims; and the family member with the strongest or most intimidating feelings generally wins.

In a permissive household, nobody ever makes an explicit distinction between feelings and facts. If Johnny, age ten, doesn't want to go to bed at nine o'clock, he should not have to do so. Johnny has a *right* to his feelings—not merely to express his feelings and to provide good reasons for them, but simply to *have* them and accept them as facts. This last is a very important distinction. All good therapists want to encourage each family member to voice his opinion; indeed, it is the lack of such communication which gets many families into trouble in the first place. But it is the mistaken assumption that *feelings and facts are the same thing* that leads many therapists, and consequently many clients, down the wrong track.

Good therapists help people understand that feelings and facts are not the same thing. If Johnny, age ten, *feels* it's unfair that he should have to go to bed at nine o'clock, his parents should ask him *why.* If he responds (with a pout), "I just feel that way," then he should be told, politely, that feelings are not accepted as facts in this household. He should be taught by his parents, with the therapist's help if necessary, that he must use his head and think of reasons why he holds the position he does.

Eventually even a "pouty" child will learn that reason transcends feelings, and that his rational judgment, rather than impulsive emotionalism, is what he needs to guide his life and get along with others.

The Child Centered Therapist

Another type of bad family therapy is child centered family therapy. Child centered, in this context, does not mean concern for the general well being of children. It refers to a consistent *bias* in favor of children against the parents. Consciously or subconsciously, such therapists assume that children and parents have a fundamental conflict of interest. And since parents are both legally and physically more powerful, the therapist sees her role as the protector of the child against the evil parents.

Evil parents undoubtedly do exist. Any social worker, attorney or law enforcement official can certainly verify this assertion. This fact explains why the state plays a role in protecting the individual rights of children against bonafide physical abuse, sexual abuse and neglect.

But one must remember that most parents are not evil; and nothing in the *nature* of the parent role gives the parent unfair power over a child. Children are, in varying degrees based upon individual ability and age, incapable of surviving on their own in the world. Until they reach physical and intellectual maturity, children need parents to handle responsibility they would not be able to handle on their own.

In exchange for this responsibility, parents must have the freedom to decide how to raise their children in the most effective way possible. Some parents are more competent than others. But all parents must be left alone to decide how to raise their children *unless* they violate the individual rights of the child through physical abuse, sexual abuse, or life-threatening neglect.

The child-biased therapist certainly believes in the rights of children; but he also brings, like all advocacy-oriented therapists, a strong personal agenda to his work. While there is nothing wrong with a personal agenda per se, since we all bring our own agendas (conscious or subconscious) to what we do, there is something wrong if the agenda involves unsupported emotional bias.

Like the militantly anti-male therapist who is quick to make snap-judgments about men, the militantly anti-parent therapist makes snap-judgments about parents. If the therapist rejects or does not understand the distinction between thoughts and feelings, for example, he will chastise parents for not treating their child's feelings as facts. If the child *feels* that his parents are mean to him, for instance, the therapist immediately puts the parents on the defensive without first either: (a) asking the child, in age-appropriate fashion, what reasons he has for feeling this way, and/or (b) asking the parents, "Is there any basis, in your opinion, for your child to feel this way?" Each of these approaches rests on the premise that feelings, however sincerely felt by a child, do not necessarily constitute facts.

On the other hand, a question like "Your child feels you're mean to him. What do you do to make him feel this way?" immediately puts the parents on the defensive and also teaches the child that he may manipulate his family (e.g., by getting them to feel guilty or ashamed) with the help of this family therapist.

Parents need to keep in mind that a family therapist or child psychologist who does not acknowledge the distinction between thoughts and feelings generally will not practice good therapeutic methods. Not only does he reinforce a seriously mistaken assumption that parents themselves may already have, but he also teaches it to the child.

Consider the case of Joe, age seven. Joe's parents experience frustration because he refuses to attend school. He says he fears prolonged separation from his parents and feels bothered by the fact that other students tease him; he also fears doing poorly in certain subjects. A therapist who utilizes the method of introspection can help both Joe and his parents see the difference between thoughts and feelings and, simultaneously, get him back to school as soon as possible so the fear does not get out of hand. Parents can be assisted in reasoning with Joe about his fear. For example:

Parent: What's your worst fear about what will happen to you in school?

Joe: That I'll fail. And that others will make fun of me.

Parent: What reason is there to think you'll fail?

Joe: I don't know. I just feel it.

Parent: Have you failed or done poorly at anything so far? Are there any facts to prove what you feel, Joe?

Joe: No. But I'm worried that I won't do well as it gets harder. Spelling and arithmetic are hard.

Parent: Why don't we wait and see? Why don't we keep talking about this, after school each day, and look and see if you're having trouble?

Joe: Can't I stay home?

Parent: No. We can talk about this, but we can't run away from our fears. Often our fears are wrong anyway. And if it turns out your fears are correct, we'll face them together and find ways to deal with them.

Without a theoretical understanding about the nature of emotions, the therapist would lean too much in either the restrictive or permissive direction. The more restrictive therapist would encourage the parents to push their son back into school right away, without providing any methods for helping Joe better cope with his irrational thoughts and assumptions. The more permissive therapist would unintentionally encourage Joe's problem by warmly sympathizing with him and, again, not providing methods for helping him to introspect and change his irrational thoughts; with such a therapist, Joe will never return to school unless forced. Many parents vacillate between the permissive and restrictive approaches.

What causes an irrational psychological agenda in the child-biased family therapist? The answer depends upon the psychological make-up and theoretical orientation of the particular therapist in question. Sometimes therapists themselves have grown up in environments where they experienced either subtle or overt mistreatment as children. Perhaps their parents used dictatorial methods and did not listen to their child's feelings. In any case, the therapist might never have considered the basic distinction between thoughts and emotions, especially if trained in graduate programs that emphasize bad forms of therapy. Consequently, many parents seek help from therapists who know as little— or perhaps even *less*—than they do about the fundamental cause of many psychological and child-related problems.

How Parents Can Minimize or Prevent the Need for Family Therapy

Using reason, parents are neither dictatorial nor permissive. Reasonable methods of raising children prevent the need for extensive mental health interventions.

Dictatorial parents apply rules arbitrarily and solely based upon their emotions. If Johnny forgets to take the trash out on a day when daddy's in a bad mood, he is grounded for a year. If the police catch Johnny shoplifting on a day when daddy happens to be in a good mood, Johnny is let off the hook. Dictatorial parents never have to explain their actions to the child. The child is to follow their rules simply because they are the parents or, as such a parent typically phrases it, "because I say so." The implication is that no better reason is required.

Permissive parents, on the other hand, allow the child's emotions to rule the house. Virtually every random feeling of the child must be acknowledged and respected. It never occurs to permissive parents—or if it does, they refuse to acknowledge it—that the child might be manipulating them. If Suzie is crying because it's bedtime, the permissive parent lets her stay up later simply to stop her crying. Or the permissive parent might insist that Suzie go to bed, but then feel so guilty about it that he caves in on some other issue at a later time. If sixteen-year-old Darrell insists that he has a "right" to his own telephone line and he begins to act up as a way to pressure his parents into agreeing, permissive parents eventually cave in just to get him off their backs. Children or teenagers who "stamp their feet" at reality are told, in effect, "There, there, let's see if we can change reality for you."

Healthy parents try to provide their children with a microcosm of a rational society. Basic ground rules are understood and enforced, rules which respect the child's age and individual personality. Only *behaviors* are subject to punishment—never thoughts or ideas, particularly if the thoughts are honestly mistaken ones on the part of the growing child.

While the responsibility rests on the kids to follow the rules, the responsibility rests on the parents to listen to their kids' grievances about the rules, provided they are rationally presented. In other words, parents should not change rules simply because a child throws a tantrum or a teenager threatens to embarrass his parents by skipping school for two weeks. In fact, parents should not even listen to a valid request from a child if it is presented in such a manner; to do so amounts to endorsing a form of emotional blackmail, thus communicating to the child that this is a valid way of doing "emotional business."

How can parents adhere to a reasonable approach in raising their children? They can begin by asking themselves: how much *freedom* and how much *responsibility* does my child currently have? The guiding principle is this: the more responsibility the child shows, the more freedom he should have; the less responsibility the child shows, the less freedom he should have. With some children, this rule operates smoothly and without discussion. With other children, unfortunately, parents must pay strict attention to this principle and never waver from it or let down their guard. If the child asks for more freedom in the absence of sufficient responsible behavior, parents need to turn the issue around. Parents need to tell the child that he cannot have more freedom until he first masters the responsibility required for his existing freedoms.

Consider, for example, the sixteen-year-old who wants to be allowed to go to a beach house with his classmates. He insists on permission to go simply because the other kids have permission. Parents need to avoid this line of reasoning; it is entirely illogical. Instead, parents must first ask themselves: Has my child been living up to his current responsibilities in a *consistent* enough way that he has *earned* such a privilege, at least for one time? The answer to this question must be thought out carefully; and it is also helpful to involve the child in this process, provided that he will not be manipulative or rude about it.

The freedom/responsibility principle applies no matter what the child's age. It becomes particularly important in the teenage years, however, because (1) the child has reached a stage in his intellectual growth where he can better match his parents' aptitude and better manipulate them; and (2) teenagers, quite understandably, are generally more demanding of freedom than are younger children; their minds and bodies are approaching adulthood but in other respects, such as financially, they are still dependent children. All normal and healthy adolescents yearn for freedom; yet parents must still set some logical limits on them, utilizing the freedom/ responsibility principle.

The principle also applies in the opposite direction. Children who accept a lot of responsibility ought to embrace a corresponding degree of freedom. If they do not, the parents should teach the child to stand up for himself and not cave in so easily to others' demands. The parent might even tell the child: "Tell me if I'm being too hard on you. I will try to watch this, but you need to help me be sure that I'm fair to you. Don't suffer silently." Despite today's media attention on the growing number of juvenile delinquents and obnoxious adolescents, there are undoubtedly still many "silent sufferers" and self-sacrificers who need their parents' attention as well.

In dealing with children, one must understand the distinction between *chastise* and criticize. To chastise a child involves condemnation of who he *is* rather than what he *does*. Chastising sends the message that the child is fundamentally worthless rather than communicating that a particular action is mistaken for a particular reason.

Chastising appears most frequently in irrational parents, although probably every parent is guilty of it from time to time. The chronically irrational parent, however, operates on the assumption that mere feelings can be facts. If his child has just done something wrong, and he *feels* at that particular moment that his child is the most evil person on earth, then to him the child is, in fact, evil. A rational parent, on the other hand, can maintain her perspective even as she feels the anger. She can recognize a child's action as wrong and tell him so without concealing her anger. But she does not let her anger by itself guide her treatment of her child in that particular moment.

Criticism means telling the child what he did wrong and *why* the adult considers the action (or idea) mistaken. It gives the child a chance to ask reasonable questions and to think over the answers on his own; he may also pout in private for awhile, if he prefers. In most cases, he will have to go along with what the parent tells him, but the parent should always be open to the child's questions and criticisms provided they are rationally presented. Even if the child has a good reason for questioning a certain rule, if he goes about questioning it in an irrational way, then the rule still applies. Emotional blackmail, or attempts to wear parents down or break their spirit, are *never* acceptable reasons for changing a rule.

Children need to be held responsible, above all, for thinking before acting. Giving in to a tantrum or any form of deliberate emotional manipulation is tremendously destructive to a child's future self-esteem; children need to learn that thinking and reasoning represent the best ways to solve problems and correct injustices.

If a child throws a tantrum, he should be humanely isolated (e.g., sent to his room or elsewhere to "cool off"). If a child tries to make a parent feel guilty for holding him responsible for his actions through such statements as, "You are a terrible mother," then he needs a calm reminder that the punishment results from *his* choices, and not the parent's. A rational parent who disciplines with his head and not on impulse can pull off this strategy with far more credibility than either the patronizing, permissive parent or the grim and dictatorial restrictive parent.

There is no substitute for a reason-based approach to raising children. My experience suggests that, if applied consistently, there will rarely, if ever, be the need for a psychotherapist. A good therapist helps the parent learn and apply this approach more consistently, if and when difficult problems arise. Since parents themselves may not have had rational childhoods, they may indeed require such help. But parents must above all understand that they *do* have the power, with practice, to raise their children in a healthy, reasonable and consistent manner.

Why Court-Ordered Therapy for Kids and Teens Cannot Work

Judges and other court officials have unfortunately adopted the same bad premises underlying bad child psychology and bad family therapy and are now applying them to the field of juvenile justice. Because the ideas of determinism, permissiveness and behavioral "disease" have become such a part of our cultural mentality, it seems unsurprising that judges and lawyers would share similarly mistaken ideas about mental health treatment.

Judges and attorneys ought to consider the perspective of a psychotherapist with over ten years of clinical experiences: *court-ordered psychotherapy is a contradiction in terms.* It does not and cannot ever work for this reason: the concept "psychotherapy"—regardless of the age of the individual being treated—implies the *voluntary* use of the client's mind or, to put it another way, the willingness to think. Thought represents the one aspect of human nature which does not and cannot respond to coercion. No one can force anyone else's mind to think.

An individual can be coerced to perform certain *behaviors,* as in the cases of slavery, paying income taxes or registering for the military draft. A mind can also be heavily influenced by powerful or persuasive ideas; but under no conditions can a mind be forced to think. The process of thought, by its very definition, requires voluntary action on the part of the individual.

Since thought does not respond to force and since, as shown throughout this book, psychotherapy involves the voluntary correction of one's logical errors in thinking, it should be clear why force and psychotherapy are fundamentally incompatible. Many will argue, of course, that offenders change their thinking when threatened by legal action (such as jail, fines, loss of property, and so on); but this view presupposes, among many other things, that criminals (even young criminals) think the same way as law-abiding individuals, an assertion unsupported by research on the subject.[65] Furthermore, court-ordered therapy jams mental health clinics with unwilling participants, taking time and energy away from therapists who can do better work with individuals who initiate the help on their own.

Instead of simply court-ordering kids to psychological treatment, judges should imply focus on *behaviors.* Judges should impose appropriately stiff sentences on juvenile delinquents, and, if they desire, encourage such individuals to seek psychotherapy when their terms are finished. The relationship between psychotherapy and juvenile justice should stop right there.

To force individuals to seek therapy is not only a contradiction in terms but can actually make matters even worse. Court officials, convicted delinquents and families are all led to believe that mental health treatment will somehow "fix" the problems which led the child to steal, assault or destroy in the first place. Parents often see the therapist as an official of the court, and transfer their resentment against the legal system onto the therapist, making any kind of collaborative relationship between parents and therapist impossible. Children in such cases may try to "con" the therapist by dutifully showing up for sessions on time and following all of the rules, thus creating the illusion that fundamental changes in their thinking are taking place.

Court-ordering children to therapy can also send the wrong message to parents of delinquents by implying that mental health professionals can take the place of raising their children for them. When these parents arrive in my office for family therapy, they are generally disappointed and even shocked to discover that the therapist's job is to hold them responsible for raising their child in the most consistent manner possible rather than simply "fixing" the problem for them. Most of the time these parents do not stay in therapy for more than a few sessions, and they fail to return my phone calls, or follow up in any way, after their premature termination. I often wonder if they go back to court and the judge simply takes their word for it that they participated in family therapy, when so far as I am concerned there never was any therapy in the first place. Is it any wonder that the proliferation of mental health services has done so little to reverse the trend of juvenile violence and family dysfunction in today's society?

Courts should stay out of the psychotherapy referral business and concentrate instead on consistent and appropriate penalties for juvenile delinquents. People who want therapy will seek it out on their own.

Diagnosis Hysteria

Another dangerous trend I have observed in contemporary child psychology involves the tendency to turn child behavioral problems into medical "diseases." Too many mental health providers appear increasingly eager to provide young children and teenagers with such diagnoses. Children who talk back to their parents or who occasionally disobey a rule are said to have "oppositional-defiant disorder." Teenagers who are truant and run away from home have "conduct disorder." If they lie, cheat and steal (or even kill) they are victims of "antisocial personality disorder."[66]

Stanton Peele summarizes the current diagnosis hysteria most eloquently: "More children are being persuaded at earlier ages that they have a disease and that this diseased person is *who* they are. We seem rapidly to be creating a future world of people who identify themselves primarily in terms of their diseases."[67]

I see evidence in support of this claim almost every day of my professional life. I encounter countless parents who have been convinced by teachers, principals and psychiatrists that their child has the disease of "attention-deficit disorder" or "learning disability," to name the two most common examples. Parents quite logically conclude that the "disease" needs to be "cured." Consequently, they fear placing any limits on their children or attempting to challenge them in any way. Even the most intelligent and well-educated parents will plead with me to explain how to "cure" their child, failing to understand the importance of teaching the child long-term goal setting, introspection and self-responsibility, the *real* tools of self-esteem.

The consequences of this cruel and unfair disease formulation extend well into the college years and undoubtedly beyond. A college teacher, for example, told me of a case where a student asked to be excused for skipping a class even though he had no good reason. His excuse? "I have a learning disability," he replied. When the teacher asked the student to explain in his own words the meaning of the concept "learning disability," the student merely shrugged, "I don't know. I was always told I had this disease and that there was no use studying; so I believed it." I sorely wish that psychiatrists and educators who flippantly hand out disease labels to the young children they evaluate would more seriously consider the long-term consequences of their sometimes ill-informed diagnoses.

Disease labels often encourage parents to ignore the fact that children can and do make choices. One of the most popular forms of labeling children is attention-deficit hyperactivity disorder (ADHD). The use of the term "disorder" implies an *inability* to pay attention as opposed to an unwillingness or refusal to pay attention. Interestingly, parents of children with ADHD frequently tell me that their kids are quite able to concentrate on activities they find enjoyable, such as music, TV, video games, or time with their peers.

According to researcher Jane Healy, research on ADHD has suggested that so far as learning is concerned, the issue is one of *selective attention*. Selective attention refers to the ability to concentrate and stay focused on a particular task, such as homework or class lectures. "But selective attention,"

Healy writes, "has proven hard to measure. Like memory, it is 'task specific,' changing according to the job the brain is asked to do and the underlying motivation to do it. For example, many teachers who complain that students can't pay attention and listen in class also notice that the same children will concentrate on a computerized video game for long periods of time. In these two situations there are clear differences between both motivational and cognitive factors such as auditory or visual attention, saliency (attention-grabbing quality) of the stimulus, requirements for memory, physical involvement, and the pace of the activity, all of which affect attention."[68] Such factors suggest that ADHD is more than a medical disease over which its victims have no control whatsoever.

The problem of disease-labeling children does not result from a shortage of government funding or well-meaning professionals. The core problem lies in the mistaken idea that behavioral problems can be labeled "diseases" in the absence of sufficient (or even *any*) physiological data, and without any reference whatsoever to the possible role of human will. Since when, you might ask, did truancy and car theft become "diseases?" Since when did manipulating parents, teachers and other authorities become a "disease?" Since when did staying up an hour past one's bedtime become a "disease?" Because there are no rational scientific principles guiding much of contemporary psychotherapy, there is no telling how far psychiatric opportunists will carry the disease concept.

Today's diagnosis hysteria can be explained by at least two specific factors. Child psychology, like all psychology, is a young science. Researchers in the field of child cognitive development are still in the data gathering stage. Consequently, psychotherapists who work with children have nowhere to turn for objective diagnostic criteria except the American Psychiatric Association's Diagnostic and Statistical Manual (known as the DSM-IV). The DSM-IV serves as a kind of "bible" for psychotherapists, including child therapists. Since the manual uncritically accepts and adopts the disease formulation for child behavioral problems, few therapists see any advantage in questioning it.

The other factor contributing to diagnosis hysteria has to do with the anxiety of parents. Parents with troubled children are naturally quite anxious. They want to apply a label to their child so they can better understand his problem and how to deal with it. It also relieves them of any responsibility in the matter. Since mental health diseases are not known to be medical problems, they do not have to feel that they passed the problem on to their child through "bad genes."

Nor are mental health diseases considered to have any remote relationship to free will—so their child need not take responsibility either. Many therapists, motivated either by a desire to reassure parents or to cash in on the disease hysteria, are quite compliant in providing parents with such labels. It is hard to imagine sending a worse message to a young child or a teenager than this: when you misbehave, it is because you are ill. Simply go to the psychologist for "treatment" and the misbehavior will stop. The psychologist will "fix" you.

Responsibility represents still another factor contributing to the labeling of children as diseased. As most Americans now realize, public schools are increasingly out of control. In more and more school districts, teachers and school officials desperately seek measures to control violent and even homicidal kids. Since many parents appear increasingly unwilling to provide even basic discipline for their children, teachers face an increasing number of behavioral problems. However well-intentioned, applying diagnostic labels to children for cognitive and behavioral problems creates the illusion that parents and children have no responsibility for the problem. Abandonment of responsibility will not solve today's growing problems in public schools.

Parents should remain wary of therapists or teachers who are in a hurry to label the child. The best therapists will want to treat child problems within a family context, and help the child return to a normal (or even better) state of functioning. The best therapists have no interest in labeling the child. Good therapists primarily want to provide parents and children with new ways of thinking and new ways of behaving so that family members can lead better lives and eliminate any genuine psychological symptoms.

Parents must also exhibit caution about a therapist who seems in a hurry to medicate the child. In my experience, psychiatric medication is rarely a requirement of good therapy for most children, and in today's climate over-medication of children is not uncommon. In many if not most cases, families and teachers need to make an honest effort at good family therapy before leaping to the conclusion that the child needs medication. Parents must guard against the ideological view of their children as victims of mysterious forces outside of their control. The child, just like an adult, has choices, and the parent's job is to teach him how to make choices consciously and wisely: in other words, to become introspective, independent and rational.

Why Good Family Therapy Is the Treatment of Choice for Most Children and Teens With a Problem

Family therapy, practiced properly, views psychotherapy as a consumer service which requires objective evaluation by the family members. In other words, the client ought to get something out of it. The therapist ought to provide the client feedback without lecturing or unsolicited advice. Good therapy seeks to solve problems rather than build a relationship between therapist and client valued solely for its own sake.

Good family therapy fulfills the criteria for good psychotherapy as outlined in chapters one and two. Family therapy by its very name suggests a contextual, as opposed to a tunnel-vision, approach. Even family therapists who see some clients individually will understand the importance of taking into account the reactions and needs of those close to the client. Family therapy also conforms to the definition of psychotherapy as an *alliance* between client/family and therapist. Good family therapy tends to focus more on the present and the future than the past.

Family therapy, despite its many strengths relative to other forms of psychotherapy, often does not place the proper emphasis on reason, introspection, and the crucial importance of distinguishing feelings from reality (and teaching children to do the same). It lacks a cognitive orientation.

Because family therapy is essentially "common sense" oriented, the better family therapists are able to send their clients in the right cognitive direction without explicit reference to the thought/feeling problem. But the fact remains that cognitive therapy and family therapy co-exist as two separate schools of thought, when in reality they are quite compatible for the treatment of children and teenagers.

Too many parents have trouble with their kids because they blindly and subconsciously follow the same emotionalist approaches to parenting that their parents and grandparents did before them. Many of today's parents grew up with authoritarian or dictatorial parents in the 1940s and 1950s. Vowing not to repeat the mistakes of their own parents, they slip into a permissive approach, often with the unqualified support of a mental health professional.

Parents who act on their feelings as if they were facts are more prone to be abusive, manipulative of, or manipulated by, their children. Once they see the errors in their mistaken assumptions and make a concerted effort to change them, emotional and behavioral change inevitably follows. Good therapists help parents discover and change these mistaken assumptions.

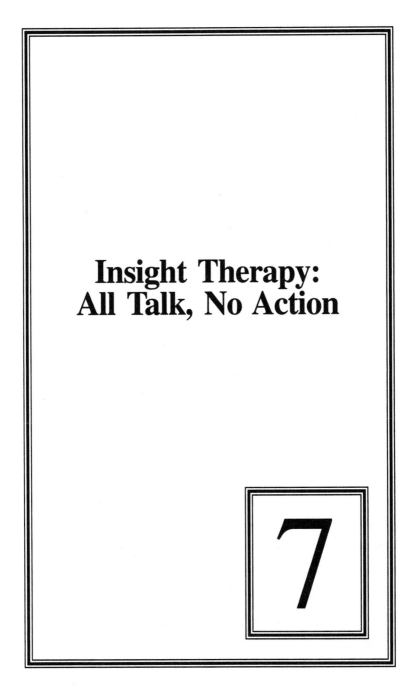

Insight Therapy:
All Talk, No Action

7

I nsight or psychodynamic therapy refers to any psychotherapy which encourages understanding about one's motives, defense mechanisms, childhood or "unconscious" without any explicit reference to how one can actually use this insight to change current emotions/behaviors in the present. Understanding the past, to the insight therapist, represents an end in itself rather than a *means* to a specific end (or goal) in the present.

Individuals typically experience insight therapy in the following way: "My therapist does not say too much. He asks me questions but he offers little in the way of feedback. And even when he does offer feedback, it's usually in the form of a question rather than an affirmative statement of what he thinks. And we spend a *lot* of time on my childhood. Even if I'm talking about a work situation, and I want a solution to the way I'm feeling about it, he tends to lead me back to my mother or father and how I felt about them. I'm frustrated. I'm not getting help for what I came in for. I don't know what this is supposed to do for me. My therapist doesn't seem all that concerned about it. It feels like we're following *his* goals, not mine."

Do such complaints mean that the therapist has no clue as to what he's doing? Not necessarily, because a therapist who sincerely believes in insight therapy thinks that by talking about the past, the client will somehow make the necessary connections to the present and feel better. Insight therapists typically assume that the client's presenting symptoms—work stress, marital conflict, family problems, anxiety attacks, depression—merely symbolize manifestations of either deeper personality problems or unresolved and "unconscious" conflicts from the client's early childhood. Insight therapy is rooted in Freudian theory which, as pointed out in chapter one, brought some very strange ideas to the new field of psychology.

Here are the basic assumptions of all insight therapies:

Premise #1: Talking can be an end in itself. Most insight-oriented therapists believe that talking about a problem can be, by itself, enough to resolve it. In one very important sense, insight therapy is on the right track. The notion of "thinking aloud" forms the basis for all good psychotherapy. Thinking aloud (or at least on paper) also serves as the basis for introspection and all cognitive therapy, as discussed in chapter three. Because so few children learn how to introspect, they grow into adults who either repress feelings or overreact emotionally.

One basic problem with insight therapy is that talking aloud cannot serve as an end in itself. It is pointless to talk endlessly about one's past without a specific purpose for doing so in the present. It is not enough to identify that a client was physically or sexually abused as a child, for example, or that her parents never encouraged her to develop her talents. One must also answer the questions: How, if at all, are these facts interfering with my functioning in the present? And what can I do to change?

For example:

Do I subconsciously approach everyone in a defensive and hostile manner, as if they were my abusive parents, thus destroying the potential for intimacy and closeness?

Do I subconsciously tend to associate with people like my hostile and insensitive parents, when in fact I should be consciously looking for individuals with different characteristics?

Do I tend to give up easily, allowing myself to be influenced by my father's idea that life is hopeless and impossible?

Do I tend to sacrifice myself for others, on the assumption that selflessness is a virtue and martyrdom is heroic? Can I reconcile the viewpoints that I should be happy, on the one hand, and that living for myself is immoral, on the other? Which is the more reasonable principle?

Good therapy seeks to link childhood to the present in direct and explicit terms, as just described. Traditional insight therapy, on the other hand, emphasizes the supposedly enormous influence one's childhood has on the present. In other words, a good therapist asks the client: What is the logical basis for this particular assumption that you hold, and how is this assumption influencing your life and emotions? An insight therapist says: Talk about the past; and talk, and talk, and talk. Reliving the past is necessary for healing your pain. Only by understanding the past can you ever change the present.

Bad therapy teaches the client how to relive his childhood as an abstract exercise, for its own sake. Good therapy teaches him to move beyond his childhood and live as a healthy and rational adult in the here-and-now.

Good therapists realize that talking is not an end in itself. Talking represents a form of communication in which talkers discuss and challenge each other's specific concepts. A passive therapist who simply listens and occasionally intervenes with subtle comments cannot do much for the client other than make her feel self-conscious and even manipulated. A therapist who understands the influence of childhood experiences on the client's thinking and behavior in the present *can* provide real help.

Premise #2: The client is the hostage of his childhood. Insight therapy, like all bad therapy, adopts the deterministic viewpoint. Determinism either states or implies that one's life is largely beyond one's control. To the insight therapist almost everything the client does is the result of unconscious childhood conflicts playing themselves out in adult life.

"Unconscious" means that such conflicts meet with resolution only through the special talents of a trained psychoanalyst. If the client feels anxious, for example, he has not recovered from a childhood desire to sleep with his mother. If a client is depressed, he may be traumatized by the fact that his mother did not breast feed him. If a client's loved ones characterize her as cheap or stingy, she may still engage in an unconscious struggle with her parents over toilet-training. If a client smokes or drinks too much, he is reacting to the fact that his parents did not let him suck his thumb long enough. Any of these explanations are possible but never ultimately provable, according to the often arbitrary nature of the Freudian method.

Rand has labeled this arbitrary approach to human motivation *psychologizing*. "Armed with a smattering not of knowledge, but of undigested slogans, [psychologizers] rush, unsolicited, to diagnose the problems of their friends and acquaintances. Pretentiousness and presumptuousness are the psychologizer's invariable characteristics: he not merely invades the privacy of his victims' minds, he claims to understand their minds better than they do, to know more than they do about their own motives."[69]

Insight therapists, although professionals and not amateurs, are the quintessential psychologizers. They exploit the desire of the masses to find explanations—*any* explanations—for their irresponsible or irrational behaviors. Psychologizers used to confine themselves to the therapy office. Today they are running amok, especially on television talk show "whine-a-thons" and amidst the rest of the intellectual rubble found on daytime television.

The insight therapist, like all psychologizers, often feels that he knows the client's motives better than the client herself ever could. Instead of actively teaching such methods as introspection so the client can better learn how to evaluate her own motives, the insight therapist is content to let her engage in a process of open-ended counseling with few (if any) explicit goals or mutually agreed upon outcome criteria.

The client who is insecure and lacking in self-esteem might enjoy this approach at first since it requires so little effort and skill. But no amount of time, expense or intellectual pseudo-sophistication can, all by themselves, help a person understand the real causes of her problems. The real causes of psychological problems are mistaken or conflicting assumptions. Sometimes—not always—mistaken beliefs develop in childhood, making it useful to look back (briefly) at one's childhood to determine the origin of these conclusions. But to spend countless hours fantasizing about how one reacted to toilet training or the sense of abandonment a client felt at the age of three when mother left father is an expensive waste of time.

Good therapists *do* believe that childhood factors influence an adult, sometimes in ways that are highly relevant to the present. But the difference between a good therapist and a psychologizer is that the good therapist can prove his case. He proves it by saying: "This is what happened to you as a child; this is what you concluded from those experiences; and this is *why* those conclusions are mistaken."

The client is free to agree or disagree with the therapist's assessment, but at least the reasons for the therapist's theory enjoy a basis in actually known facts. The insight therapist has nothing better to offer than arbitrary and often bizarre ideas about the client's childhood, purely abstract theories (i.e., all toddlers are sexually attracted to their parents) requiring blind faith since they have no known connection to reality.

Premise #3: A lack of focus is not only acceptable—it's desirable. Perhaps the best method for unmasking a true insight therapist is to say the word "focus." Watch his eyes glaze over in horror as he shifts uncomfortably in his chair.

The insight therapist understands what the concept *focus* implies. It implies responsibility on both the client's and therapist's part to determine what the purpose of therapy is to be. It requires specific, *objective* terms and concepts. It requires that the therapist earn his $100 per hour. It requires that the therapist do something other than nod, make ironic comments and occasionally ask, "What do *you* think?"

Insight therapy presumes that psychotherapy is an open-ended process which must be long-term in nature (usually years) and completely subjective with respect to the criteria for beginning and ending therapy. "Subjective" means that when it *feels* like time to start therapy, it *is* time to start therapy; and when it *feels* like time to end therapy, it *is* time to end therapy—unless the therapist feels otherwise, of course. No other reasons or explanations are necessary, although they might or might not be provided depending upon the particular therapist.

I remember once interviewing a woman who had spent the last ten years in insight therapy.

"Has it been helpful?" I asked her in our first session, scheduled because of problems she was having with her daughter.

"I never asked," she responded.

"Is the therapy working?" I persisted, incredulous.

"I never thought about it that way."

"What kind of feedback has your therapist provided you?" I asked.

"Very little. Except that I am not ready to stop."

In insight therapy, open-endedness represents an end in itself. No objective basis exists for either beginning or ending therapy. Some insight therapists believe that therapy should continue for one's *entire* life, or at least for several decades. Altogether evaded or unacknowledged by the insight therapist are the basic facts that: (1) feelings alone are not a guide to proper decision-making; and (2) for any human endeavor to be successful, all parties must understand, in as explicit terms as possible, what the purpose of the endeavor is and how they will know when it reaches successful completion.

Insight therapists often disregard the fact that some life problems *can* be quickly resolved. Sometimes solutions *are* simple. Most important, insight therapy cannot be successful since no criteria of success are ever defined. Of course, therapy without objective criteria cannot *fail* either; perhaps this fact explains why psychoanalysis subsisted as a cash cow for so many years. Without an expected outcome, sadly, psychotherapy is nothing more than an expensive process of emotional and intellectual masturbation— often more for the therapist than for the client.

Premise #4: Everything is a disease. Insight therapy rests on the grossly mistaken assumption that problems of mood, behavior, judgment, and even morality all constitute forms of *disease.*

Examples abound. An hysterical woman is not being irrational, according to insight therapists; she is a victim of "histrionic personality disorder." A stressed-out yet conscientious and hard-working businessman is not simply in need of a rest; he is suffering from "narcissistic personality disorder." An obnoxious, overbearing and demanding self-victimizer is not simply immature and irrational; he is afflicted with "borderline personality disorder." An aggressor with violent outbursts who destroys property is not a criminal; he is the tragic victim of "intermittent explosive disorder."[70] The disease formulation knows no limits.

None of this should be construed as a denial of the fact that many individuals have serious psychological problems. What needs correction is the mistaken premise that the emotional consequences of illogical thinking can be considered medical diseases. Most emotional and behavioral problems without a known biological base are due to basic errors in thinking.

If John assumes he has a right to be loved, for example, then it is entirely logical that he beat up his wife when she falls out of love with him; assumptions cause emotions.

If Sue believes that children have a duty to live for their parents, then it is certainly appropriate for her to feel depressed when her son drops out of college and joins the air force because he longs to fly; beliefs cause emotions.

If Bill thinks that unconditional love is enough, by itself, to change his girlfriend's basic personality, then it is absolutely normal for him to feel frustrated and confused when she is exactly the same two years later; what one thinks determines what one feels.

Probing the childhoods of John, Sue and Bill will not change their emotional states; probing—and changing—their thoughts and beliefs *will*.

It is only by identifying cognitive errors, contradictions and misunderstandings and developing methods to correct them, that psychotherapy can be of any use. Such errors can only be corrected by the willful efforts of the individual who makes them, whether a therapist is part of the process or not. Involving a good therapist in the process facilitates (or speeds up) the process, but in the end only the *individual* can change his mistaken assumptions.

The *Un*conscious versus the *Sub*conscious

As stated throughout this book, part of evaluating one's therapy involves assessing the theories and premises underlying the therapist's approach. Insight theory utilizes the Freudian notion of an unconscious. According to classical Freudian theory and most contemporary insight-oriented psychotherapy, the unconscious represents an entity with a will and purpose of its own, both unknown and entirely outside the control of one's conscious mind.[71] The unconscious rules our behaviors and actions in ways which we cannot ever hope to understand—except, somehow, by engaging in endless years of psychotherapy for no specific purpose with little or no explicit feedback from the psychotherapist.

I advise rejecting the use of the concept "unconscious" in favor of the *subconscious*. The subconscious mind simply refers to that which you are not focused on at any given moment. An analogy of a computer screen may be helpful here. All computers contain a data memory stored on a disk. The disk is your subconscious. It contains all the date, files, programs and other information previously entered (through experience and learning) into the data base (one's memory). The computer screen is your conscious mind. Since the screen is limited in size and scope, there is obviously only so much information which can be viewed on a screen at any one time. The same is true of your conscious mind.

The subconscious mind does not have a will or life of its own. In fact, there is nothing in the subconscious which was not originally acquired by *conscious* means. When a person stops thinking about something, that material (i.e., idea, emotion, conclusion, assumption) goes from the conscious to the subconscious mind.

The subconscious is responsible for the automatic performance of emotions—some of which are logical, and some of which are not. The conscious mind is capable of both knowing and, when necessary, changing what is in the subconscious mind.[72] This is both the value and the goal of good psychotherapy: identifying the hidden premises in one's troubling emotions and determining whether or not they are logical.

Insight therapy rests on precisely the opposite view. Insight therapy is based upon the old Freudian idea of unconscious.[73] According to the Freudian view, the unconscious engages in self-generated cognitions which are extremely difficult, and perhaps impossible, for the individual to access without the long-term help of a psychoanalyst. The conscious, rational mind has little control over the unconscious world. People have no choice but to accept this fact and suffer through years of unfocused insight therapy.

In some respects, the Freudian idea of unconscious is similar to the religious notion of "soul." Just as the believer can only be forgiven and cleansed of his sins through the mystical grace of a priest, the analytic client can only reach "insight" through the remote guidance of a trained insight therapist. There is precious little difference, in fundamental terms, between the medieval confessional and the contemporary office of the insight or psychodynamic therapist. Each requires penance: one moral, the other financial.

A Case Study: Insight Therapy

Viola P., a thirty-year-old unmarried woman, has a problem with food. She eats too much. She has eaten too much for most of her life. Despite an otherwise attractive appearance, she is more than one hundred pounds overweight. Her friends tell her she should try to lose weight. She has tried many different diets. Some of them work, but only in the short-run. She loses ten or even twenty pounds, but experiences a setback and then is back to her old eating habits again, worse than ever. She has a satisfying professional life and a number of wonderful friendships with both men and women. But she has no sex life and has no apparent prospects for a happy marriage because of her size. She decides to seek the help of a psychotherapist.

Dr. I. is an insight therapist. He practices insight therapy in its undiluted form. "Undiluted" means he consciously and explicitly accepts the four major premises of insight therapy described in the previous section. He begins therapy by doing a thorough family background assessment of Viola. This assessment lasts for approximately ten sessions. In addition to asking for basic medical and family history, Dr. I. probes for many more details than Viola expects. He asks for her earliest childhood memories and even tries to put her under hypnosis (unsuccessfully) to help her remember details prior to the age of two. He wants to know at what age she began toilet training and for how long it lasted. He wants to know similar facts about each of her four siblings.

He wants to know at what age her parents married, and he wants detailed descriptions of the growing up experiences of each of her parents.

During the eighth session Viola politely asks Dr. I. why they have not yet dealt with her specific eating problems. She points out that after having spent nearly $1,000 she would have expected at least to have made some progress. In reality, she has actually gained another ten pounds since her first therapy session. The doctor points out, a bit sharply, that therapy is not a "quick fix" and Viola should not expect to have her problems solved overnight. Viola quietly accepts this argument, although inside she still has some doubts and even anger about her therapy. She feels that her question was reasonable, but she also assumes that the doctor must know what he's talking about. So she continues with the therapy.

In the tenth session, Dr. I. generously provides some feedback to Viola. He tells her that she is still engaged in an "unconscious struggle" with her mother. He has determined that as a child she competed with her mother for her father's affection. Although her father did give Viola attention, he could obviously never be her sexual partner. This led Viola to be a rather withdrawn and depressed child. Her mother, sensing this fact and also busy with raising other children, tended to comfort Viola with food. This subtle pattern enabled her mother to feel less guilty for her victory over her daughter in the sexual competition with her husband, and it tended to make Viola feel better as well. Dr. I. tells Viola that there are many other complicating factors and that it will require several years, at least, of intensive therapy for her to "work through" her issues of conflict with her mother, as well as to identify sources of conflict with other family members.

Viola leaves the tenth session with mixed feelings. On the one hand, it was nice to receive some concrete feedback from Dr. I. after having so far spent $1,000 for her treatment. On the other hand, she is discouraged to find that she will have to spend thousands of more dollars before she gets well. She is not sure what Dr. I. means by "working through" and "unresolved unconscious issues." She is also disturbed by the fact that Dr. I. does not even attempt to address the ongoing problem of her weight, the most important issue in the here-and-now.

At the next session she tells Dr. I. her concerns. She reminds him that since the beginning of therapy she is actually eating more, and not less. She asks what signs she should look for during this long period of treatment to indicate that she is on the right track. Dr. I. seems a bit perturbed by her questions. His irritation is noteworthy because he normally does not show any kind of emotional reaction whatsoever. "Therapy is not designed to treat symptoms," he says. "Therapy needs to treat root causes. Perhaps your tendency to focus on symptoms is an unconscious defense against the hard work you know is ahead of you in therapy. It will not be easy to work through all of the unresolved conflicts you have with your mother. And who knows what other things we will find. Consider this carefully," he frowns. "You cannot escape these conflicts. You will never deal with your eating unless you first resolve these other conflicts."

Viola remains unconvinced. But she also feels that she has no choice but to continue. This man would not hold his degree if he were not competent, she reasons; and the state would certainly not license an incompetent therapist.

In subsequent sessions, she is simply encouraged to talk freely about her childhood. There is no specific focus to any of the sessions. If she has nothing to talk about, her therapist asks her questions about her childhood or continues a discussion from an earlier session. If she has a session on a day when she is particularly agitated about something—

for example, an incident with a co-worker or a fight with a friend—she is helped to probe her "unconscious" for indications that she is "projecting" her unresolved feelings towards her mother onto these individuals.

Viola finds therapy to be an interesting, and at times intriguing, exercise. But she continues to overeat. At one point she loses four pounds, and she hopes that the therapy is finally taking effect. But sure enough, she returns to her old habits and gains back another seven pounds. She seems stuck in the same old pattern of gaining, losing and regaining weight. She holds out hope that somehow, over time, the good doctor's treatment will relieve her of her problems.

Analysis: Viola's therapy rests on all four of the premises of undiluted insight therapy. Talking is treated as an end in itself. If Dr. I. has some purpose in asking Viola the questions he does, she does not understand its nature. If she confronts him with the gap between her goals and what the therapy seems to be accomplishing, he treats her very reaction as an "unconscious" defense mechanism which must somehow involve her mother. Dr. I.'s feedback and treatment plan portrays Viola as a hostage of her childhood, the alleged sole cause of her current problems, and as the victim of a personality "disease" rather than simply holding mistaken, habitual assumptions which she can actively and consciously change. The sessions are deliberately unfocused as the therapist allows them to drift indefinitely.

A Case Study: Good Therapy

Renee L., a thirty-year-old unmarried woman, has a problem with food. She eats too much. She has eaten too much for most of her life. Despite an otherwise attractive appearance, she is more than one hundred pounds overweight. Her friends tell her she should try to lose weight. She has tried many different diets. Some of them work, but only in the short-run. She loses ten or even twenty pounds but experiences a setback and then is back to her old eating habits again—worse than ever. She has a satisfying professional life and a number of wonderful friendships with both men and women. But she has no sex life and has no apparent prospects for a happy marriage because of her size. She decides to seek the help of a reputable psychotherapist, Dr. C.

Dr. C. identifies himself as a cognitive therapist. He operates on the assumption that emotions are consequences of subconscious assumptions or premises. He assumes that the primary goal of psychotherapy is to help an individual discover the cause of his irrational behaviors or emotions and seek to correct the problem through "restructuring" of basic, relevant premises.

Dr. C. begins therapy by doing a thorough assessment of Renee. He asks questions about family background, but he also asks her questions about her basic values and ideas. In the evaluation he discovers that Renee has a high regard for work and career but often feels that because she is so career-oriented she cannot find a man with whom to share her romantic life and possibly raise children. She knows that this is illogical, but she has to admit to feeling this way a great deal of the time.

In the first session, Dr. C. asks Renee to identify what she would like to see happen as a result of coming to therapy. He encourages Renee not to worry about how long therapy will take; instead, he tells her simply to focus on what she wants to see change.

Renee finds this a provocative question, and instantly senses the importance of answering it carefully. In attempting to answer the question, she gradually starts to realize that she wants to change both the way she eats and the way she looks at herself. She wants to learn to eat in order to stay alive and not to meet complex emotional needs. She also wants to learn why she continues to overeat despite the fact she knows it's both irrational and unhealthy.

She and Dr. C. reach an agreement to work for ten weekly sessions and then reevaluate. Dr. C. cautions her that there are no "miracle cures" for overeating, and she obviously will not lose all the weight she desires in a mere ten weeks. But he also says that they both should be able to identify evidence that the therapy is working at that point, to perceive concrete examples that she is headed in the right direction. As a first homework assignment, Dr. C. asks Renee to keep a daily log of her feelings, with special attention to what she feels just prior to having a snack. Dr. C. stresses the importance, for the time being, of trying to monitor her feelings when she desires to eat rather than eliminating the behavior itself.

Renee leaves her first session feeling hopeful. She had not expected her therapist to be so open and responsive. She had always heard that therapists can be aloof and suspicious, and it was a relief to find a therapist who was warm and personable. She enthusiastically begins to keep her journal. Although Dr. C. told her not to concentrate on dieting for awhile, she discovers that by making herself write down her feelings whenever she craves a snack, she tends to eat less.

Over the ten weeks she makes some fascinating discoveries, some of which her therapist points out and many of which she sees on her own. She learns that she tends to eat whenever she worries about a meeting at work the next day. While she always knew such meetings made her nervous, she did not realize they were a factor in her compulsive snacking. Her therapist encourages her to identify her fears about the meetings and to question their validity. For example, she questions her assumption that it would be the "end of the world" if she made an error in her weekly presentation at the meeting. Honest mistakes, her therapist suggests, need not necessarily be disasters. To experiment with this theory, she intentionally makes a small error at the next meeting and discovers that, through making a joke about it, she puts both herself and her colleagues more at ease.

In the first ten weeks she also learns an important reason why her childhood had an effect on her current eating patterns. As a child, she was taught by her mother to be an independent and career-oriented woman. While she is grateful to her mother for teaching her how to cope in the world on her own, without having to depend on a man for financial survival, she also recognizes that her mother had difficulties accomplishing this goal on her own. Her mother tended to cope with the stress of being independent and career-oriented in the 1950s by relying on food as a way to calm her nerves. Fortunately, her mother never developed a weight problem because of physiological factors which enabled her system to break down calories more quickly. Unfortunately for Renee, she inherited her father's metabolism which led her to gain weight more easily than her mother ever would.

Through a process of introspection taught to her by Dr. C. in their eighth session, Renee discovers the reasons why she does not have to repeat her mother's tendency to cope with being a career woman by overeating. First of all, she reminds herself that she is now in a cultural climate where most assume that women will pursue careers, while in the 1950s the opposite was generally true. Secondly, her mother could afford to use food as a coping mechanism because her body had a very different metabolism. While the bad news remains that she cannot eat as liberally as her mother, the good news is that she has the incentive to pursue more healthy and rewarding outlets. She decides to join a gym and work out three times a week, along with moderating her intake of food high in calories and fat.

At the end of ten sessions, Renee has lost ten pounds. Although she is still very overweight, both Renee and her therapist see objective evidence that she is on the right track. She has developed new thinking habits which have led to different behaviors—namely, less snacking and more exercising. She has also discovered a very mistaken assumption behind her irrational feeling that she cannot be both a career woman and a happy individual with a fulfilled romantic life. While she knows there is still much work to be done and a lot of improvement to be made, she feels less pessimistic about the prospects of losing weight. The greatest help of her therapy, she feels, is that she is now more in charge of her life. She understands that her assumptions affect both her emotions and her behaviors, and only through identifying and changing her mistaken assumptions can she expect any other kind of change.

She and Dr. C. conclude that her therapy has been helpful. Because she has more goals to work on—her struggle with occasional anxiety attacks, for example—she and Dr. C. make a contract to work together for another ten sessions. They agree that during this time Renee will continue to exercise and keep her "snacktime" journal of feelings. Dr. C. also gives her some assigned reading on anxiety and during the sessions they both work to identify mistaken assumptions which might be revealed during her anxiety attacks.

Renee is not sure how long she will need to be in therapy. Dr. C. encourages her not to dwell on this fact. He reminds her that the important issue is that she continue to work on identifying and changing her mistaken ideas and that she should continue in therapy only so long as there is a need to do this and she finds the sessions helpful. Renee feels comfortable with this plan and decides not to worry. She is too busy making psychological changes she never thought were possible.

Analysis. The contrast between good and bad therapy should be striking. Therapists such as Dr. C. practice all of the basic characteristics of good psychotherapy. The therapist provides feedback on a regular basis. The client utilizes therapy as a vehicle of empowerment to change herself, not simply become bogged down in despair and bad memories. She learns how to conform her feelings to the facts and not simply complain when the facts fail to conform to her feelings.

The therapy is clearly problem-focused and solution-oriented. Renee's immediate environment (e.g., snack habits, exercise of lack thereof) is taken into account. She is neither encouraged nor discouraged by her therapist to discuss the past; the past is integrated into the present only when necessary, as is the case when she identifies her childhood conclusion about the impossibility of becoming both a career professional *and* someone with a fulfilled personal life. And, last but not least, the therapeutic relationship is one of alliance: therapist and client work together on a problem without losing perspective of the fact that, in the end, only Renee can identify and change her unhealthy methods of thinking. Renee is left to feel more responsible for her life even as she receives warmth and support from a therapist who seems to care about helping her become well.

The Hazards of Insight Therapy and Psychodynamic Theory

Frustration. One potential consequence of prolonged, unfocused insight therapy is frustration. The client might feel that she has more understanding about her past but lacks any clue about what to do next. She understands that she felt left out and ignored as the middle child, but she is no closer to resolving the interpersonal conflict she has with her boss or her teenage daughter than when she first entered therapy.

Because the insight therapist is often passive and quiet, there is an aura of mystery and authority about the therapist which many clients find too intimidating to confront. Consequently, they sometimes seek out a different therapist. They may approach the new therapist with suspicion, dread and even hostility. They are beginning to wonder if psychotherapy is not simply a waste of time, while simultaneously wanting to give another therapist a chance. They *want* to focus on a goal and take responsibility for their lives, yet they also want to talk with someone who is genuinely compassionate and will not approach them as if from a remote throne in the sky. I encounter such insight therapy dropouts on a regular basis.

For those who stick with insight therapy for a long time, the consequences become even more devastating. Consider adults who were genuinely victimized as children, perhaps through physical, sexual or objective emotional abuse. Good therapy encourages such individuals to view resulting emotional pain in adulthood as the consequence of mistaken conclusions—e.g., "The world is a dangerous and hostile place in which everyone is out to exploit me"—which can, with effort, be corrected and changed in the present.

Insight therapists take a different approach. The insight therapist wants the client to dig deeply into the past, far more than is necessary for resolving whatever is wrong in the present. It is thought that this will somehow resolve unconscious conflicts of which the client is neither aware nor capable of controlling.

Helplessness. Insight therapy ignores the idea of human volition. Volition refers to the fact that as a human being— a thinking, creative animal—one is capable of making choices and accepting responsibility for those choices by learning from mistakes and always seeking to improve oneself. Volition represents the most important aspect of human consciousness and human psychology: the power to discover the causes of emotions and to change them, when necessary, through the use of thought.

If insight therapy ever accomplishes this goal, it does so only by accident, or else because the therapist accepts some of the premises of good therapy while rejecting some of the more dangerous premises of insight therapy. But pure, consistent insight therapy is anti-volitional, as is any psychotherapy rooted in Freudian ideas.[74]

According to Freudian theories, human beings are helpless creatures caught up in a jungle of unconscious conflicts beyond their control. Consequently, Freudian therapists teach their clients to rely on the therapist rather than on themselves, an approach entirely necessitated by the depraved view of human nature to which they subscribe. If man is nothing more than a beast waiting to happen, after all, then why wouldn't he need a therapist to cling to for the whole of his miserable existence?

According to Freudian theory, man, if left to his own devices, would devour the world in a rage of uncontrolled aggression and sexual desire. As one critic put it, Freud saw man as little more than "an excrement-molding pervert itching to rape his mother."[75] In order to keep these instinctual urges under control, says the Freudian, psychological defenses develop within the human psyche. Supposedly, only a psychoanalyst or insight therapist can uncover the role that psychological defenses play in our everyday lives and problems.

Psychoanalysis is a process of five, ten or even twenty years in which one must place a great deal of faith and trust in both the analyst and the therapeutic process itself. And if the client experiences doubts along the way, the analyst has a smug answer for all of them. If the client becomes distressed that therapy is not helping, he is accused of "transferring" his anger at his mother (who rejected him in favor of his father) onto the therapist. If the client is late for an appointment, it must signal an indication that she is transferring other childhood anxieties onto the therapist. The possibilities are as limitless as the imagination of the therapist, and as bottomless as the client's pocketbook.

Irrationality. The primary flaw of psychoanalysis and insight therapy, which is simply watered-down analysis, lies in its deprecation of human reason. While claiming to rest on scientific principles of logic and rationality, psychoanalysis actually influences one to develop a highly irrational approach to life. Instead of emphasizing responsibility for one's own life and actions, it encourages an almost unbelievable dependence on the therapist for a prolonged period of time. Instead of allowing the individual to identify and learn to introspect about the origins of his feelings, the analyst takes it for granted that feelings have causes in unresolved childhood conflicts beyond the adult's ability to control or change, at least *consciously.*

The insight therapist relies upon a peculiarly circular form of logic. Consider an example to illustrate this point. A twenty-two-year old man seeks the help of a Freudian insight therapist. He is experiencing depression over a recent breakup with his girlfriend. The therapist tells him, after several sessions, that the young man's depression represents a resurgence of feelings of abandonment he felt as a child. The break-up with his girlfriend merely triggered feelings of depression, which existed unconsciously long before he even met the woman. Once he met this woman, he unconsciously transferred the unresolved feelings of abandonment onto her. Thus, the real cause of his depression is not the illogical assumption that his girlfriend represents an irreplaceable loss;

the real cause is the fact that he has unresolved feelings of abandonment toward his mother. In order to "work through" this underlying "abandonment issue," he needs to attend therapy on a twice weekly basis for an indefinite period.

The man replies that he recalls no such feelings of abandonment. In fact, both of his parents were always very supportive without being too intrusive as he became older. He even has many warm memories of his mother and father taking him to the park as a young child. He certainly feels abandoned now, in the present, because his girlfriend has left him. In fact, one of the reasons he finds it so traumatic is that he never has really experienced abandonment before; the loss of romantic love scares him to death, because it represents such a new feeling.

The insight therapist goes on to explain that all young boys go through a period of "competition" with their father for their mother's affection. Normally, of course, the child loses this contest and inevitably feels a sense of rejection as he gradually comes to this realization. He cannot have his mother to himself; ultimately he must accept that his mother belongs to his father. When the girlfriend cuts him off, he relives the feelings of abandonment and experiences depression because he does not understand the origin of those feelings.

Why does the young man not remember any of the abandonment he felt from his mother's sexual rejection of him? Because, according to the insight therapist, he was so young and because the process was unconscious.

Would his father or mother remember any of this psychodrama, since they were older? No, because the process was unconscious for them too.

What then is the proof of this theory of human "psychosexual" development? It is to be found, the insight therapist believes, in the writings of Sigmund Freud or perhaps the neo-Freudians.

How did Freud discover these facts since they are unconscious to all parties involved and therefore nobody remembers them? "Through the process of psychoanalysis, when they come out in symbolic forms, such as free association of emotions or dream interpretation," the Freudian true believer will respond.

And on what basis does one conclude that emotions or dreams represent unresolved abandonment issues from childhood? "Why, Freud's theories and research, of course," says the analyst.

What if the young man concludes that this theory is pure hogwash and that insight therapy will not be helpful to him? He must be unconsciously transferring the rage he felt towards his father as a young child onto the therapist. Perhaps the young man is not an appropriate candidate for analysis, the therapist might sniff, although he is strongly advised to "resolve" these issues involving his father.

All of this exemplifies a circular form of reasoning. No proof exists for Freudian theory, because no proof is possible. In fact, Freudianism does not, strictly speaking, constitute a "theory" since proof is irrelevant to its formulation. Freud's "theory" of psychosexual development springs from the free associations (i.e., feelings) of his clients. Analysis of the free associations, in turn, arise out of the interpretations he makes from his theory. Without reference to the free associations, no theory is possible; without reference to the theory, the free associations remain meaningless.

Nobody can prove that young boys want to sleep with their mothers and fear castration from their fathers because, the Freudians claim, these emotions are inaccessible to one's awareness except through the special, almost mystical graces of a psychoanalyst. Insight therapy relies upon faith in Freudian theory and the special, yet never explicitly defined, healing powers of the psychotherapeutic process. In scientific terms, it remains about as effective as prayer.

Purposeful Purposelessness. Unlike most other forms of therapy, insight therapy is explicitly open-ended. In other words, it is without goals or focus *on purpose.*

Most of us assume that goals are important. If we want to be happy in life, we must have goals: to become a carpenter, a teacher, a financial wizard, an engineer, an architect, to raise children, or, presumably, to become a happier person. It seems reasonable, therefore, that seeking out the help of a professional also involves some kind of goal. We hire accountants to help with last year's taxes. We hire a physician to help cure, if possible, a medical complaint. We hire an auto mechanic to install new brakes. Should a psychotherapist help a person achieve some specific goal as well?

The stale defense that "human psychology is not that simple" does not justify years or even decades of unfocused, insight-oriented therapy. Of course human psychology is not simple. This truism explains why so much demand exists for psychotherapy in the first place. But precisely how does it help people to make their lives even *more* difficult by telling them they are at the mercy of unconscious emotional conflicts beyond their ability to solve logically?

Is therapy to address only symptoms (i.e., feelings) rather than causes (i.e., thoughts/assumptions)? If psychotherapy is indeed a science, then its practitioners should make use of whatever knowledge exists to help their clients discover how to cope with reality. A prospective therapy client should expect nothing less.

The concept of "insight" implies new knowledge or understanding about some topic—in this case, possible explanations for one's motives and behaviors. Hopefully, insight represents an ongoing phenomenon in all of our lives. It is not necessary to engage in five or ten years of psychotherapy to become insightful. One can gain insight so long as one is conscious and alive, with or without the help of a therapist. Nor should insight stop simply because psycho-therapy has been terminated.

Malevolence. Because of the influence of Freudian think-ing, prolonged insight therapy can lead to a sense of ma-levolence and anxiety-ridden pessimism.

Think about classical Freudian theory and all that it im-plies regarding human nature. From the very beginning of life, the child is thought to be engaged in a state of almost constant psychological and sexual warfare with his parents. If in everyday conversation an adult says something stupid or out-of-context—a "Freudian slip"—it is automatically as-sumed that there is some hidden and diabolical message from the unconscious contained in the statement.

Self-confident individuals, according to Freudian diagnoses, are "narcissistic," simply because they do not project the im-age of low self-esteem that all normal, depraved human beings ought to project. Quiet and introspective individuals are con-sidered "avoidant" simply because they choose not to go along with the crowd. And virtually everything that an adult says, thinks or does is reducible to something that happened in the first three years of life. Under the Freudian philosophy life becomes a psychological minefield in which every phrase, thought and behavior must be ruthlessly dissected and filtered through the malevolent premise that man is—by nature—an irrational, devious and sexually repressed animal.

No wonder such therapy needs to go on for years and years.

The most psychologically dangerous aspect of malevo-lence lies in its self-perpetuating quality. The more one accepts the idea that man is helpless and irrational by nature, the more dependent one becomes on authorities to be told what to do.

Or, put another way: The more a client works with an insight therapist, the greater the need to continue seeing the therapist. If Jack first goes to a Freudian therapist with the idea that he has some problems but they can probably be worked out, and that such problems are ultimately under his control, he will have a very different idea after a year or two of insight therapy. He will probably have a sense that life is so complicated that he will never be able to undo all the damage from childhood—but thank goodness he has the therapist to talk to every week. "What would I do without my therapist?" is the prevailing attitude of such individuals.

Something is seriously wrong if a therapist either directly or indirectly encourages a client to think this way. My experience with numerous psychodynamic colleagues suggests that too many of them have a malevolent view of human psychology; irrational Freudian theories have led them to believe that all human beings are helpless, depraved creatures ruled largely by glands and emotions. I do not recommend putting the precious trust of one's very soul into the hands of an individual with this view of human nature.

Philosophies such as Freud's, which cannot be proved or disproved by logic, are eventually abandoned by reasonable thinkers and left with tradition-bound enthusiasts to carry on in their wake. The longer such philosophies last, the more passionate and rigid the successive generations of their proponents become. For this reason, we can expect insight therapy to be around for a long, long time despite its notorious ineffectiveness, and despite the increasing unwillingness on the part of health insurance companies to finance it. Freudianism is dying, but it will probably never die out altogether.

Let the buyer beware.

How to Avoid Hazardous Insight Therapy

Once again, the state of the psychotherapy profession can lead to discouragement. How is one to distinguish between a malevolent insight therapist and a therapist with a better view of life?

The client should take responsibility for setting goals prior to the first therapy session and then asking the therapist for help in achieving them. A true insight therapist will recoil at this approach. He will try to discourage the client from setting concrete goals and instead place the emphasis on early childhood development at the expense of everything else in the here-and-now. Try to find a therapist with a cognitive orientation, or at least one who seeks to help set realistic, objective goals.

Remember that insight does not represent an end in itself. It is not true that only long-term, open-ended therapy can discover causes of psychological problems. Emotional dysfunction is the result of mistaken or distorted assumptions. The real cause of psychological problems is distorted thinking and automatized beliefs unsupported by the facts of reality. Only by changing these assumptions—with or without psychotherapy—can a person hope to earn an improved emotional state. A good therapist can help a client discover irrational, automatized assumptions as early as the first session.

Childhood, per se, does not cause emotional problems. Mistaken conclusions often formed in childhood can lead to later problems. Therapist and client should only discuss childhood to discover distorted thinking habits or false generalizations still held, however subconsciously, in the present. Discussing childhood ad nauseam, for its own sake, is of no value at all. In fact, it can actually lead to an increased sense of self-pity, hopelessness and helplessness. I regularly see clients victimized by such an approach.

Don't let it happen to you.

Behavioral Therapy:
We Are All Robots

8

Behavioral therapy refers to any psychotherapy which rests on the assumption that individuals feel and act the way they do solely (or mostly) because of conditioning or training by others. Behavior therapists emphasize the characteristics human beings share with animals and altogether ignore that which is crucially and uniquely human: our capacity to think and make choices independently and with the use of reason.

Human beings differ from animals in their ability to form abstract concepts, which are the vehicles of rational thought. Abstract concepts do not merely apply to the domain of scientists and other intellectuals. All conscious human beings—even uneducated ones—are by nature *conceptual,* rational animals. Nonhuman animals do not share with humans the ability to conceptualize. Ayn Rand has distinguished between the perceptual level, which humans share with higher animals, and the conceptual level unique to humans:

> As far as can be ascertained, the perceptual level [of young human beings] is similar to the awareness of the higher animals: the higher animals are able to perceive entities, motions, attributes, and certain numbers of entities.

> But what an animal cannot perform is the process of abstraction—of mentally separating attributes, motions or numbers from entities. It has been said that an animal can perceive two oranges or two potatoes, but cannot grasp the concept "two."[76]

What exactly *are* concepts? Concepts are generalizations which allow human beings to retain a wider and more sophisticated range of knowledge than animals could possibly grasp. Once a child mentally grasps the concept "table," for example, he is able to retain this concept each time he encounters *any* flat, level surface with support(s). The child, once having learned the concept "table," retains the notion of "flat, level surfaces with support(s)" each time he encounters a new table.

A dog, on the other hand, can only recognize any one individual table by its perceptual characteristics: size, shape, smell, color, location, and so on. If you get rid of your familiar kitchen table and replace it with a new one, the dog will not instantly recognize it as another instance of the concept "table"; he will simply recognize it as another object with a different shape, size, color and smell.

Human beings are capable of forming concepts; nonrational animals are not. Concept-formation is what distinguishes the rational animal from lower species. We humans are rational animals because we form concepts. Concepts represent the basis for all of our communication, inventions and technological wonders. And our ability to form concepts is, ultimately, our means of physical and psychological survival.[77]

Of course, the very notion of concepts implies a distinctively human, rational mind to engage in the cognitive process of concept-formation. Theorists such as B. F. Skinner, who originated behavioral therapy, found both concept-formation and, by implication, the human mind to be inconvenient to their goals.[78] According to the behaviorists, human beings are composed of (1) physiological/biological matter, and (2) actions or behaviors. These two factors represent the sum total of a human being. What we commonly refer to as "the mind" or human consciousness amounts to nothing more than a series of biochemical reactions. We humans are presumably nothing more than animals with a different physiological structure and a different way of behaving. The fact that as a species man has progressed from the cave to the computer microchip, while all other forms of animal life are limited to the same predetermined biological behaviors year-in and year-out, receives no attention from the behaviorists.

One psychologist summarizes the behaviorist position in this way:

> Behaviorists define psychology as the study of "observable behavior" (their term for action) and claim that man's behavior is controlled by the environment. In *Beyond Freedom and Dignity,* Skinner states that "a person does not act upon the world, the world acts upon him." Thoughts do not cause actions, according to Skinner, but are simply another type of behavior: "covert behavior." Learning is not defined cognitively (as the acquisition of knowledge) but as a change in behavior, caused by the environment. Behaviorism dispenses with such concepts as the self or personality, emotion, and mental illness, and replaces them with behaviorally defined notions such as response repertoire, bodily reaction, and abnormal behavior.[79]

Even if one knows little about psychology, or the types of philosophical generalizations from which all psychological theories arise, the psychotherapy consumer must have some understanding of what behavioral theory really means. Behavioral theory denies the phenomenon of human choice. Every behavior and every thought is the product of factors in the environment. Every move one makes, every word one utters, every "original" idea which enters one's mind, amounts to nothing more than a response conditioned by various stimuli in the environment: church, media, schools, parents or whatever. One cannot control one's mind or life; the average human is every bit as intellectually helpless as a pet dog, cat or fish. People are determined *strictly* by biological and social forces in the environment and history. Period.

As these views illustrate, behaviorism represents deterministic philosophy taken to its ultimate limit. According to behaviorism, human beings cannot assume responsibility for their behaviors or emotions; each person is determined by forces outside of his control.

Behaviorism, in its undiluted form, is the theory upon which an Adolf Hitler—or any totalitarian dictator—can rely in rationalizing a warped, inaccurate view of human nature. Strict behaviorists ignore the facts that: (1) *thinking,* not behavior, is what distinguishes human beings from all other animal life; and (2) thinking is a purely voluntary, *self-generated* process which can only be performed with the individual thinker's full participation and consent.

These facts do not negate the influence of the opinions and actions of others in the environment. But neither do they deny, as the behaviorists do, that all individuals are free to change their opinions either through a solitary process of introspection or the results of another's introspection which they *independently* assess to be correct.

Thinking, in the end, is an entirely individual process which only the individual thinker can generate. Otherwise, how could B. F. Skinner have developed his theory in the first place? He would merely have been the product of various stimuli in his environment, thereby making his theory (and *all* theories) incapable of being independently, rationally judged as true or false.

Behavioral therapy teaches the individual that he is a product of everything around him except his own conclusions and value judgments. Left out of this idea is any indication of how human beings have surpassed the achievements of all other animal species who, unlike humans, engage in the same biologically predetermined behaviors day in and day out for hundreds, even thousands, of generations at a time.

Behavioral theory rests on the premise that there are no essential differences between humans and animals. In accepting such a view, the client's psychological status is reduced to the level of a salivating dog. Once one understands that behaviorism is a hopelessly irrational philosophy of life, one will start to see why behavioral therapy amounts to a counterproductive method of mental health treatment.

The extent to which the behavioral therapist practices behaviorism in undiluted form is the extent to which such therapy must be considered psychologically toxic. The behavioral therapy client must realize that he participates in a process which operates on the world view that human beings are essentially animals. In a field generally thought of as "humanistic," this concept seems the most anti-human idea imaginable. Such anti-human ideas cannot solve psychological problems in any long-term way.

To help illustrate this point, consider the following case examples.

Behavioral Therapy and the Tantrum-Throwing Child

Mrs. K. takes her five-year-old son to a behavioral therapist. She is frustrated because her son throws temper tantrums on a regular basis. If she tells him to brush his teeth, he throws a tantrum. If she asks him to wash his hands for dinner, he throws a tantrum. If she asks him to sit quietly in the waiting room while she gets her hair cut, he throws a tantrum. Because of all the media attention on attention-deficit and conduct "diseases," Mrs. K. assumes that her son needs medical treatment. Her son's pediatrician, however, refers her to a behavioral therapist instead.

The behavioral therapist asks Mrs. K. very detailed questions about the events surrounding each of her son's tantrums. For example, he wants to know exactly what Mrs. K. does after each tantrum incident. Does she ignore it? Does she try to appease it? Does she punish it? It is difficult for Mrs. K. to answer these questions accurately, so she follows the therapist's advice to keep a daily log. After reviewing the log for a two-week period, she and her therapist discover that she has been—however unintentionally—*rewarding* her son's tantrum behavior. In order to get him to quiet down, she offers him food or appeases him by compromising her position (e.g., "OK, Johnny, I'll let you stay up another fifteen minutes past your bedtime—but that's it!")

The behavioral therapist makes the following recommendation: From now on, Mrs. K. is to pay special attention to how she responds to her son's tantrums. She is to avoid rewarding or appeasing his behavior in any way. When he throws a tantrum, she must immediately punish him in some way. This might involve making him sit in a "punishment" chair or in a corner for a specified period of time. It might involve taking away a special treat he would normally receive in the absence of a tantrum.

In order to cure the behavioral problem, says the therapist, one must treat the symptoms. The symptoms (i.e., the tantrums) can be controlled through effective behavioral management. Nothing more or nothing less is required. Therapy should aim simply at "what works" in controlling the behavior, within reasonable limits. There is no need to even address the notion of cause.

What is wrong with the behaviorist's approach? In one sense, nothing. He is correct that Mrs. K. is, without realizing it, appeasing her son's behavior by not taking a firmer stance. Her son, unlike other children, probably requires a very black-and-white approach to discipline, at least until he demonstrates greater self-restraint without the need for punishment. And the behaviorist is also correct in asserting that consequences for one's actions must be considered as part of the therapy process. His approach is based upon logical scientific observation, as his request that Mrs. K. keep a two-week log suggests.

So where's the problem? The strict behavioral therapist, as opposed to the *cognitive*-behavioral therapist (as cognitive therapists sometimes call themselves), ignores the fact that all human beings must think. He ignores the fact that man does not live by behaviors alone. All human beings, including young children, need to understand the reasons for a particular behavior. The following example illustrates how this principle may be applied to the misbehaving child.

Adult (to child): Why are you sitting in the corner?

Child: Because mommy punished me.

Adult: Why did mommy punish you?

Child: (Pause) Because I wouldn't come to dinner when she asked.

Adult: So. . . . You *chose* not to go to dinner when mommy asked, and now you have to sit in the corner.

Child: I guess so . . .

Adult: I'm sorry you're going through this. But maybe some good will come out of this, as a learning experience. Maybe you'll learn to think more carefully before you make such choices in the future. Think how much better you'd feel right now if you had only made a different choice.

This example illustrates that behavioral factors such as discipline, while crucial, are not the sole conditions governing human (including child) behavior. Choices, even bad choices and not carefully thought out choices, are still choices. Choices do not originate in behaviors but in actual thought processes within the individual human being. Furthermore, this principle applies both to children and adults. Children must learn to understand the concept of "choice" at an early age along with rational introspection. Punishing them will not, by itself, teach them how to think.

Behavioral therapies can be seductive, especially to parents who want a quick-fix for a difficult child. The danger of behavioral therapy, however, lies in its failure to recognize the importance of the human mind, even in a young child. Granted, a five-year-old mind is in many respects an unsophisticated one. But it does not change the fact that a human child has the capacity to reason, even if on a less sophisticated level than an adult. To emphasize reward and punishment in the absence of attempting to reason with the child on his or her own level, is to ignore a critical aspect of human psychology. It sends the message to the child, however unintentionally, that rules and authority are all that matter in life. Independent thought, with the use of logic, is downplayed or even condemned.

Pure behavioral therapy can also reinforce the mistaken assumption shared by many over-stressed parents that disciplining a naughty child is all that matters. Such a mistaken assumption can, in extreme cases, set the stage for physical abuse. If discipline is all that matters, the logic goes, then it must be OK to beat a child into submission if he does not follow rules the first or second time.

In my opinion, behavioral discipline only works as a consequence of a child's clear choice not to listen to reason. Punishments should always be preceded by one (and generally only one) warning to the child of *what* the consequence will be if he fails to act properly and *why* it is important that he act properly. When possible, the child should be given a chance to ask reasonable questions about the rules and why they are being applied in a particular case. Whenever a parent punishes a child, he should point out to the child that the punishment resulted from his own failure to think. For more details on reasonable ways to raise kids, see chapter six.

Behavioral Therapy and a Compulsive Eating Problem

Barry L. eats too much. He is thirty pounds overweight and, at the age of thirty-five, is concerned about the potential for high blood pressure and even a heart attack. On the advice of a friend, he decides to seek the help of a behavioral therapist so that he can learn to control his eating habits.

In the first session the therapist asks Barry to carefully log the times and places that he eats—particularly snack times, since these are the times when he eats compulsively.

After examining the log in the next session, the therapist notices a very clear pattern in Barry's eating habits. Barry apparently overeats only when he has a very stressful day at work. Since his job is stressful by nature, he compulsively snacks on more days than not.

The therapist prescribes the following: Barry is to find a new method for dealing with his stress. Instead of compulsively eating, he will develop the habit of running each day after work. Over time, according to behavioral theory, he will substitute the habit of snacking with the habit of running as a method of coping with stress.

What is wrong with this approach? Nothing—so far as it goes. Exercise can be a useful and certainly much healthier substitute for snacking. It just seems like common sense. Unfortunately, the behavioral therapist completely ignores the role of thinking in the development and maintenance of Barry's compulsive behavior. Behaviors are often the consequence of an individual's emotions. Emotions, in turn, are caused by thoughts and assumptions. The behavioral therapist fails to recognize that Barry's real psychological problem is not the eating per se; the eating is really a consequence of another factor: his subconscious assumptions and evaluations.

What are the subconscious evaluations and assumptions of a compulsive eater? The possibilities vary from one individual to the next. Perhaps Barry has made the assessment that he must have constant control over literally *all* aspects of his life, from the weather to the opinions of others. Since such an unrealistic view naturally creates internal conflict, he finds that stuffing himself with food temporarily relieves that conflict in a pleasurable way.

Another possibility is that Barry sees himself as invincible, and thinks that he should be able to eat all he wants even though it clearly must have long-term health consequences.

Still another possibility is that Barry, because he has always been such a hard worker, has never learned the importance of finding relaxing activities for himself. He assumes that a hard worker does not and should not require leisure time; and when he does find himself with free time, it makes him feel guilty. Instead of enjoying his free time, he berates himself for it. His compulsive eating, then, arises out of the self-destructive assumption that leisure time is intrinsically bad and wasteful.

Behavioral therapy would never have explicitly addressed any of these problems. Learning to "associate" running with stress instead of eating with stress, thereby changing his behavior, does nothing to address what caused Barry's behavior in the first place: his thoughts and assumptions.

A good therapist would, first of all, probably have seen that Barry needs to get in better touch with his feelings. He would have instructed Barry to keep a journal of what his feelings were immediately prior to his snacking. Since feelings are psychological "printouts" of one's subconscious thoughts and assumptions, this journal would have provided the therapist with some clues as to the origin of Barry's compulsiveness.

If therapy does not first acknowledge the role of the client's thoughts and emotions, then it is impossible to have any kind of long-term impact on one's behaviors. Even if behavioral therapy "works" for Barry, he will simply replace one form of compulsion with another. Instead of being compulsive and guilt-ridden about eating, he will become compulsive and guilt-ridden about running. If it rains, he will become angry and frustrated because he cannot run. If he misses a day for a good reason, he will berate himself for not being invincible. Or if he evaluates himself as an inadequate runner, he might give up in disgust and return to compulsive eating simply because it feels good.

Unless he learns to (a) identify and (b) consciously change his mistaken assumptions, Barry cannot be helped by psychotherapy—at least not over the long-run. To encourage Barry simply to replace his snacking with running might seem like common sense. Unfortunately, doing something healthy for the wrong reasons is little better than doing something *unhealthy* for the wrong reasons.

The Hazards of Behavioral Therapy

Control by Others. Behavioral therapy can lead the client to feel like a "puppet" of the environment. "What I do depends on where I am. If I want to stop gossiping, I need to stay away from Mary. If I want to stop overeating, I need to stop going to restaurants. If I want to curb or eliminate my drinking, I must not even associate with people who drink responsibly. If I want to be less depressed when I'm at home, I need to divorce my husband and move far away."

While sometimes one does, after careful thought, need to change one's environment for specific and logically valid reasons, a solution does not always require such a change; and it certainly is not the *first* alternative, as behavioral therapy leads one to believe. As already discussed, introspection comes before behavioral change.

Lack of Self-Responsibility. Behavioral therapy also implies a far more destructive notion, an idea which is strangling contemporary society: that an individual is not responsible for any of his or her actions. Behavioral therapists will deny this charge, but the premises of their approach logically *must* lead to an approach to life which encourages irresponsibility.

The client who takes behavior therapy seriously can tell himself: "If all of my emotions and behaviors are the product of forces outside of my control, and if my rational mind is powerless to change my thoughts and behaviors, then I must not be responsible for any of my actions. If I can't control my emotions and behaviors, then how can I be responsible for them?"

Narrow-Mindedness. Like all bad therapy, behavioral therapy also represents a "tunnel vision" approach. The classic example involves the behavioral therapist or psychiatrist who sees only the mother and child in the sessions, ignoring the influence of the father and other family members.

Unless the family is comprised solely of mother and child, this approach can be futile and unfair. Even from a purely behavioral perspective, the therapist, concerned with rewards/punishments and nothing else, is incapable of understanding the full context in which the child lives without the participation of all adults raising the child. Even if the father is absent, there could be other significant family members (grandparents, unmarried romantic partners, siblings) who participate in and in some way comprise part of the family system.

It saddens me to see mothers dragging their mentally "diseased" children into mental health clinics to talk to the therapist or psychiatrist without the father or other relevant family members ever being involved. What kind of message does this send to a child who is already growing up in a society where fathers are often not held accountable for their responsibility in child rearing? And what message does it send to fathers, who might want to be involved but assume the therapist does not care if they participate?

Ignorance of the Past. Behavioral therapy, unlike the insight therapy approach, is often praised for focusing on the present. Indeed it does. At the same time, behavioral therapy is guilty of sacrificing the past to the present. Good therapy does not ignore the past. It simply seeks to point out mistaken conclusions from the past, where relevant, in the present.

Good therapy neither dwells on the past (as insight therapy does) nor completely ignores the past (as behavioral therapy does). It seeks to integrate the past into the present by identifying both the accurate and inaccurate conclusions an individual has formed in his life so far.

Anti-Reason, Anti-Intelligence. Altogether disregarding the need for reason, behavioral theory assumes that human beings just engage in certain behaviors; no further explanation is necessary. A man goes to work because he is conditioned to do so by the society in which he lives. A child studies in school because he is conditioned to do so by his teacher. Einstein developed his revolutionary theories because he was conditioned to do so by the environment in which he lived. Period. The same presumably applies to all the geniuses and monsters of human history, famous or infamous.

Behaviors without reference to cognition, choice and individual initiative hardly constitutes a basis for human psychology.

Simplistic. Behavioral therapy is sometimes thought to be the "common sense" psychotherapy. It flourished in the 1940s and 1950s as a reaction against decades of seemingly senseless insight therapy. Since insight therapy dealt with vague, abstract issues which could only be fully "understood" by the trained analyst, behavioral therapy provided a language and set of principles which clients could be expected to understand as well.

While insight therapy was unfocused and impractical, behavioral therapy sought to establish itself as scientific and practical. While insight therapy could take forever, behavioral therapy sold itself as remarkably short-term. While insight therapy was largely subjective, behavioral therapy represented the supposedly objective alternative.

Many good, rational psychotherapists feel attraction to behavioral therapy as an approach. Such therapists sincerely want to practice a treatment approach grounded in reality and intellectual consistency—two qualities for which insight therapy is not well known. I personally believe that for these good intentions such therapists are to be applauded.

At the same time, once again, good intentions do not guarantee good therapy. If a therapy relies upon mistaken premises then its potential to create positive changes disintegrates. Where many well-meaning behavioral therapists go wrong is in their assumption that common sense is enough upon which to base a science of psychology. It is not. If psychology is a science of human beings, then the distinctively *human* capacity for thinking and reasoning, as opposed to merely sensing and perceiving, must be taken into account.

Common sense is helpful at the perceptual level, but a *science* requires the help of the more generalized, conceptual level of human capacity. Otherwise, there would be no justification for a psychotherapy profession in the first place. Reason, because it integrates large amounts of sensory evidence into conceptual abstractions, represents a more sophisticated form of human thought than mere common sense; it enables a therapist to give clients general principles ("Only become romantically involved with someone who shares your values") rather than simplistic, concrete-bound advice ("Leave the bum"). Consequently, good therapy cannot and should not ignore reason.

Denial of the Subconscious. Behavioral therapy denies the existence of a subconscious, where one's underlying assumptions and ideas are held in storage.

As an example of how the behavioral therapist ignores the subconscious, consider this strictly behavioral assessment:

"Joe grew up in an unhappy family. Now as an adult he is depressed. Why? Because he was conditioned to be depressed by his depressed parents, who were in turn conditioned to be depressed by *their* depressed parents. The only way to break the cycle is to put Joe in a setting where he will not be exposed to any depressed people."

This solution might sound reasonable, but it leaves unanswered many important questions. What kind of generalizations did Joe form as a child which led him to grow up to be depressed? What errors in thinking does he now make which lead him to make bad choices in the present? What is the best way to convince Joe of the need to learn introspection so he can identify his mistaken assumptions through logic and gradually work on changing them? What are the *choices* Joe can make for himself in order to alter his emotional state?

The need to answer these questions presumes that (1) Joe has an independent, volitional consciousness; (2) Joe, while influenced by his depressed parents, is capable of identifying and thereby changing his mistaken assumptions; and (3) Joe is not a helpless creature of the environment which conditions him. These are three points the cognitive therapist makes. (The better cognitive therapists makes them explicitly; the less sophisticated ones, implicitly).

The behavioral approach, if accepted by Joe, could lead him to follow a significantly different course of action than the cognitive approach. If he accepts the behaviorist's premise that his feelings are determined by others in his environment and not by his *own* method of thinking, then he might hastily decide, for example, to divorce his depressed wife. Yet what if his wife is not aware that she is depressed? Is there no way to convince her? And if she becomes convinced, can she not also overcome her depression by becoming more introspective and changing her mistaken assumptions?

Ideas Matter

Remember that the theoretical approach of the therapist, to whatever extent the client adopts and absorbs it, will influence the way the client makes major life decisions in the future.

Before making any major decisions while in psychotherapy, the client should identify the views of the therapist she sees. If the views are behaviorist in nature, and suggest that unhappiness is caused exclusively by one's environment and behaviors, and not at all by one's convictions, then the client should think carefully before allowing the therapist to influence her decisions.

Clients should also remember that the good therapist is not a determinist. The rational therapist assumes that one's assumptions and ideas underlie all emotional states. While such assumptions can be difficult to identify, and often do require the help of a good psychotherapist, at least a person can consciously choose to change the way he thinks and acts.

Finally, therapy clients ought to keep in mind that behaviors are caused, ultimately, by thoughts and choices. Behaviors are sometimes indirectly caused by emotions or by undue influence from other individuals or institutions (family, parents, the media, and so on.).

In the end, nothing changes the fact that an individual remains free to think differently using an independent and self-generated process of introspection. While this process can be difficult and will sometimes fail, the fact that all human beings possess a capacity for reason cannot be ignored.

Mystical Therapy:
Where All Feelings
Are Facts

9

Mystical therapy represents the umbrella term for any psychotherapy which rests on the *explicit* suppositions that (1) more than one reality exists, and (2) the means for accessing other "realities" involves either a special individual (such as a psychic or priest-equivalent) or one's raw, unexamined emotions (or a combination of both). In short, mystical therapy refers to the twentieth-century version of black magic.

Why address such practices in a book on psychotherapy? In fact, why even dignify them with the term "psychotherapy?" There are two reasons.

First, these are not the only forms of bad therapy which rest on irrational assumptions. Other forms of therapy, such as insight and behavioral therapy, also exhibit a complete or partial ignorance of the role of human thinking in the maintenance of psychological health. In a sense, mystical therapy represents a more honest form of the methods which behavioral and insight therapists disguise under the pretense of "science." Most bad therapists preach the virtue of rationality and introspection while practicing methods based to a large extent on emotionalism. Mystical therapists drop the pretense and simply preach and practice emotionalism outright.

Secondly, I see everyday evidence in my practice to suggest that more and more otherwise rational individuals are placing trust in such methods. A young woman, for example, becomes stuck when trying to determine a career change. When I ask her to explore her feelings aloud, she informs me that she saw a psychic who told her there would be a major career change in her thirty-first year. It makes her uncomfortable to contemplate a career change while she's only twenty-six because it may somehow interfere with her "fateful" choice to be made five years in the future.

Intellectually, this client agrees with my suggestion that anything which happens in the future can only be the product of choices made in the here-and-now; yet she clings to the psychic's prediction on the premise that "she [the psychic] might be wrong, but she might be right as well."

Feeling, usually quite accurately, that conventional psychotherapies have failed them, believers in mystical therapy might come to the conclusion that they need something different: something *radically* different. They want a simple answer, and they want it now. Who better than a psychic, a mystic or some other figure to provide them with what they are convinced they cannot discover themselves through reason, observation, and introspection? How better to escape from responsibility and independence than relying on a fortune teller?

James Hillman:
A Case Study in Mystical Psychology

It is important to understand that mystical therapy, despite its anti-intellectual assault on the most fundamental tenets of science and reason, has been inspired by the ideas of highly respected psychologists. James Hillman, author of *A Blue Fire* and various other works, serves an excellent example of one such psychologist.

Hillman and like-minded advocates of mystical therapy advocate a new way of thinking about mental health treatment. They ask clients to give up the "fantasy" of cure, repair, growth, self-improvement, understanding and well-being as primary motives for psychological change.[80]

Instead, they ask clients to surrender their conscious minds to blind emotions and to wallow in such emotions for their own sake. Psychic "healing," channeling, and reincarnation "regressions" are among the recommended methods for reaching the mystics' vague goal of "higher consciousness," their term for improved mental health. Irrational as these approaches may sound, Hillman and other mystical therapists enjoy the admiration and love of a growing number of therapists and clients alike.

Unlike their more hesitant colleagues in the Freudian, neomystical schools of thought, mystical therapists drop all pretense at attempting to sound rational, scientific or in any way connected to reality. In this respect, at least, they must be credited for their uncompromising consistency.

Mystics reject the very concept of a volitional, thinking consciousness and replace it with the religious notion of a "soul" completely detached from the body. The religious view assumes that body and "soul" (i.e., mind, consciousness) can be completely detached, while the non-religious view sees the mind and body as interconnected. Instead of helping their clients integrate the mind and body so that thoughts and feelings are in harmony, mystics deliberately seek to disintegrate any hope of connection between thoughts and feelings. In so doing they leave individuals with nothing to act on *except* their feelings since there is no hope of ever attempting to discover objective truths about one's own life or life in general.

What is the nature of insanity under such a view, a view which overtly denies the existence of objective truth? On this point Hillman leaves little doubt as to where he stands:

One day in Burgholzli, the famous institute in Zurich where the words *schizophrenia* and *complex* were born, I watched a woman being interviewed. She sat in a wheelchair because she was elderly and feeble. She said that she was dead for she had lost her heart. The psychiatrist asked her to place her hand over her breast to feel her heart beating: it must still be there if she could feel its beat. "That," she said, "is not my real heart." She and the psychiatrist looked at each other. There was nothing more to say. Like the primitive who has lost his soul, she had lost the loving courageous connection to life— and that is the real heart, not the ticker which can as well pulsate isolated in a glass bottle.

This is a different view of reality from the usual one. It is so radically different that it forms part of the syndrome of insanity. But one can have as much understanding for the woman in her psychotic depersonalization as for the view of reality of the man attempting to convince her that her heart was indeed still there. Despite the elaborate and moneyed systems of medical research and the advertisements of the health and recreation industries to prove that the real is the physical and that loss of heart and loss of soul are only in the mind, I believe the "primitive" and the woman in the hospital: we can and do lose our souls.[81]

The second paragraph is an especially good illustration of the notion of subjectivism. Subjectivism, in this context, refers to the idea that one way of looking at things is no more or less valid than the other. Hillman actually claims that the psychotic client's delusion is no more or less valid than the psychiatrist's objective assessment based on the use of his reason and sense organs. Furthermore, like all mystics, Hillman detaches human consciousness (the "spirit") from the body, assuming one must choose one or the other: he assumes one must settle for being either a sensitive soul out of touch with reality, or a reality-oriented hardhead without sensitivity or "soul." In short, one must become either a fool or a louse.

Objective reality either does not exist or is impossible to know, according to the mystical view. Only unsophisticated, judgmental anti-intellectuals would dare to claim otherwise. Yet if this is so, why do we even have a psychotherapy profession in the first place? Why spend thousands of dollars paying a therapist such as Hillman to "heal" a client if no objective basis exists (or *can* exist) for judging that something needs to be "healed" in the first place?

Furthermore, why is Hillman's "reality," as presented in his books, any more or less valid than anyone else's; and if it is not, then what business does he have making authoritative assertions in the first place? If Hillman's line of reasoning is taken to its only possible conclusion, one is left with nothing but an endless loop of circular logic and, psychologically, hopelessness and despair—which, as will soon be seen, Hillman considers to be moral virtues rather than psychological problems.

One should not, of course, ignore the perfectly valid use of metaphor, either in therapy or in the more traditional arena of the arts. It is possible, for instance, to speak of a "broken heart" due to the death or loss of a loved one without meaning the literal rupture of the organ inside one's chest. Imagination and creativity *are* perfectly compatible with sanity and mental health, contemporary "art" forms notwithstanding.

But subjectivists and mystics do not merely defend the use of poetic metaphor as a means of adding a romantic, happy, "soulful" dimension to the often harsh reality of life. Mystical subjectivists seek to obliterate the very idea that any rational means exists for knowing *anything,* thereby reducing the human mind to a mass of consciousness and emotions with no connection whatsoever to objective existence. Given their subjective premises, mystics are logically consistent in concluding that mental illness is a myth and that no one person's "reality" is more or less accurate than another's.

The entire therapeutic philosophy of mystics rests on the illogical assumption that the only *correct* way to view reality is through an acceptance of the idea that no correct way exists. Notice the self-refuting contradiction here? There are no absolutes except, of course, for the mystic's *absolute* rule that there are no absolutes.

Notice, too, Hillman's moralistic attack on the "elaborate and moneyed systems" of the medical profession. One wonders if he would be quite so judgmental if *he* were on the operating table of a brain surgeon, or being treated in an emergency room after an automobile accident. Would Hillman truly want to be treated for massive head wounds and internal injuries by a physician who does not believe that the real is the physical? Would he trust a brain surgeon who told his assistants, in effect: "Do what's right for you. Brain surgery means different things to different people. Your reality will tell you one thing; mine may tell me another."

Would the mystic trust the pilot of an airplane on which he was a passenger to adopt the view that no "correct" or "incorrect" method exists for landing a jet? If not, then why is human consciousness—or what Hillman and other mystics refer to as the "soul" or "spirit"—any less reliant on objective standards?

Mystical therapists, like the Freudian neomystics, take it for granted that human nature is fundamentally and necessarily at war with itself. In psychological terms, this assertion means that thoughts and feelings can never be in harmony. The mind, or one's consciousness, can never be in harmony with the body, one's material existence. The conscious, rational aspects of man can never hope to integrate with the subconscious, automatized ones. The purpose of psychotherapy, from the mystical perspective, amounts to the disintegration of consciousness, or the total divorce of reason and emotion. The client becomes healed *not* when his emotions and rational thoughts are integrated, but only when his consciousness breaks apart through "dismemberment."[82]

Just as mystics deny the possibility of harmony between reason and emotion, they also glorify depression and other mental disorders as an accomplishment. Mystical therapists do not merely state that depression, while a painful and undesirable state, can often be a useful tool for resolving subconscious psychological problems. Hillman, so typical of the mystical therapist, goes one step further and proclaims that depression itself *is* a desirable state.

"Depression is essential to the tragic sense of life," he writes favorably, thus implying that a tragic sense of life, as opposed to an optimistic and hopeful one, represents the essence of mental health.[83] Keep in mind that Hillman is the hero of many contemporary psychotherapists who are supposedly "treating" their clients for the very problem of depression he claims is so desirable!

Hillman's other assaults on human nature make the delusions of Freud, Skinner and others seem shallow by comparison. He says that a major goal of psychotherapy involves creating a state of mind no longer concerned with the difference between appearance and reality.[84] He actually considers depression a morally superior "achievement" precisely *because* of the depressed person's inability to distinguish between feelings and reality. Instead of seeing depression as an undesirable state, Hillman sees it as a desirable state *for precisely the reasons it ought to be considered undesirable.*

As a mental health professional seriously committed to helping individuals discover the joy and challenge in living, I find it difficult to dignify something so profoundly irrational with any further comment. Hopefully, the delusional nature of mystical psychology speaks for itself.

Mystical Therapy and the Hazards of Accepting the Arbitrary

Mystical therapy, grounded in mystical theories such as Hillman's, amounts to an unapologetic glorification of the subjective. Feelings are not merely seen as a wonderful part of life; feelings are seen as the *only* means of making assessments. Raw, unexamined emotion is all that counts.

Mystics actually condemn the introduction of rationality into the therapeutic process. Rational introspection is the furthest thing from a mystical therapist's mind. In fact, the idea of distinguishing between thoughts and feelings probably never occurs to the mystical therapist, or if it does, he will dismiss anything related to thinking as inappropriate for therapy. If the good therapist relies on the principle "think your way to the truth," the mystical therapist relies on the opposing principle "feel—and only feel—your way to whatever you feel like."

Not all mystical therapists are self-anointed priests and psychics. Some mystical therapists even have medical degrees. One particularly respectable form of mystical therapy is hypnosis. First, an important distinction must be made between mystical hypnosis and rational hypnosis. Rational hypnosis presumes that hypnotic techniques are simply a means of helping an individual relax or learn to focus better on one particular issue in his life. A good therapist might teach the client hypnotic techniques, for example, as a method of quitting smoking or controlling compulsive behavior. While I personally question the long-term effectiveness of such methods for most people, these hypnotherapists do not necessarily violate the critically important scientific principles that (1) there is only one reality, and (2) that reality can only be understood through the independent use of one's reasoning mind.

Mystical hypnosis, however, involves an assumption on the part of the therapist that the hypnotic state is somehow another dimension of reality where hidden truths and memories reside. Most mystical hypnotists rely on the Freudian notion of the unconscious (see chapter seven) in making this claim.

Mystical therapies use the Freudian unconscious to justify completely bizarre and arbitrary claims in ways that Freud himself undoubtedly never intended. Some mystical therapists, for example, claim that we are all reincarnated souls from previous lifetimes. How do they support such an unfounded assertion? Simply by claiming that one's dreams and unconscious images reveal memories from past lifetimes. If you have a dream about falling off a cliff, for example, this means that you died in a previous lifetime by falling off a cliff. If you have the same image during a hypnotic "state," the same interpretation will be made.

In addition to arbitrary hypnotic interpretations, other typical examples of mystical therapy, besides irrational hypnosis, include the following:

(1) "Out-of-body" regressions, where one's consciousness is thought to literally "leave" the body; these are done for one of many purposes, including a "return" to a previous lifetime or attempting contact with an all-knowing or all-powerful Deity;

(2) Suspension of consciousness, where one deliberately stops thinking altogether. While meditation can be a very helpful relaxation tool, mystical therapy clients learn it as a way to "check out" of reality rather than as merely a means of relaxing and helping to better focus on goals;

(3) Primitive therapy, such as listening to a beating drum so one can better access one's "inner" or "transpersonal" self;

(4) Dream analysis in which dreams are viewed as access to other levels of reality rather than merely a state of pre-consciousness in which fragments of one's subconscious form what are likely random associations with one another; and,

(5) Spiritual therapy in which the "spiritual guide" is a psychic, medium or some other individual appointed to guide you to another plane of existence or consciousness.

Consider the similarities between the mystical and the Freudian approaches by using a brief analysis of a dream about falling off a cliff. Granted, the Freudian analyst might interpret the dream in a different way than the mystical therapist. He might say, for example, that the cliff represents the mother's vagina, and that the guilt associated with secretly wanting to sleep with one's mother leads to an unconscious association of sexual desire and death.

The Freudian, wearing his scientific robe, would probably scoff at the mystic's supernatural claim of "past life" memories. Yet neither the mystic *nor* the Freudian has any evidence to support his claim other than through his arbitrary theory. The Freudian starts with the unproven and unprovable premise that all toddlers want to have sexual intercourse with their opposite-sex parent. This premise is then used as a basis of everything else, including the interpretation of one's dreams. The mystic, on the other hand, starts with the unproven and unprovable premise that we are all reincarnated souls of earlier lifetimes. This premise is then used as a basis for everything else, including the practice of past-life regression.

The basic error made by both the Freudian and the mystic is identical: each fails to recognize that facts *do not* arise out of theories. On the contrary: *theories arise out of facts.* One cannot arbitrarily assert—in the absence of any hard, observable data—that all toddlers want to sleep with their parents and then develop a sweeping theory of human nature on that base. Nor can one arbitrarily assert—in the absence of any hard, observable data—that all human beings are reincarnated souls and then develop a psychotherapeutic method on that base.

In all fairness, the Freudian at least makes some effort to connect his otherwise arbitrary theories to the fields of science and introspective observation. The reincarnation therapist, on the other hand, literally devises his claims out of thin air. This attribute distinguishes a totally off-base mystical therapist from a merely misguided, inaccurate Freudian therapist.

A client who wishes to avoid the hazards of mystical therapy needs more than simple common sense. A client must first learn something about the way real scientists think. Real scientists do not accept arbitrary claims. An arbitrary claim is one for which no observable evidence exists. Consider the following exchange:

Tom: That blue jay in your back yard is the reincarnation of Elvis Presley.

Sue: (Startled). What? Are you crazy? What makes you say this?

Tom: Because we are all nothing more than souls reincarnated from one life to the next. We can even be a different species across lives—a bird in one life, a man in another, a woman in still another.

Sue: But how can you prove this?

Tom: (Condescendingly). How can you disprove it?

Sue, although certain she is right, is helpless to respond. This is because she does not understand the importance of rejecting the arbitrary. The full definition of the arbitrary is as follows:

> An arbitrary claim is one for which there is no evidence, either perceptual or conceptual.
>
> It is a brazen assertion, based neither on direct observation nor on any logical inference therefrom.[85]

Sue's response to Tom's outrageous claims should have been like this: "Your point is not valid. You are the one making the claim, so you are the one who has to provide evidence for it. Your feelings do not count as evidence. Until you show me evidence, I do not have to consider your claim one way or the other."

If somebody makes an arbitrary assertion—either in the realm of science or the realm of everyday life—it is not your responsibility to discover ways of refuting it. The burden of proof rests with the individual who makes the claim in the first place. Until he can provide evidence that his claim is true, you are in no position to argue in any way.[86]

Consider an example of an arbitrary assertion in connection with psychotherapy:

Wife: (To husband) I feel that you are in a state of denial about your work addiction.

Husband: Why? What makes you think I have a work addiction?

Wife: Denial is a psychological process in which the individual refuses to acknowledge his sickness. Just by asking me these questions you are proving that you're work addicted. Your defenses are up; you don't want to consider the ramifications of your disease. You have, as my therapist has told me, a narcissistic personality. You are selfish and wrapped up only in your concerns. You're in denial.

Husband: I am not selfish! I resent your therapist making diagnoses of me, having only met me one time. Who does she think she is? I just like my work. And you wouldn't own all the nice things you have if it weren't for my high-paying job. Including that pricy therapist you see!

The husband's reaction, while perhaps understandable and valid in this context, nevertheless reflects a basic error:

accepting the arbitrary. His wife has accused him of having a "disease" without providing any sensory or logical evidence for her assertion (other than the alleged authority of her therapist). Her claim, therefore, represents an assertion of the arbitrary.

When anybody, whether a scientist or a spouse, makes an arbitrary assertion, the listener *must* remember that he is under no obligation to argue. Until, or unless, the asserter provides evidence which may then be either refuted or conceded, it is impossible to argue. And it is very bad for one's case to become defensive, as the husband did in this example. A better and more appropriate response would have been as follows:

Husband: You are placing me in a lose-lose situation. If I argue with you, then you'll accuse me of denial, which is part of the "disease" you mention. If I walk away and say nothing, you'll accuse me of the same thing. Therefore, I simply refuse to respond to what you're saying. When you offer evidence to support your claim, we can talk. But until then, you haven't shown me anything.

This issue involves far more than abstract philosophy and logic. It is an issue of profound importance in the lives of everyone. Both men and women of varying degrees of intelligence and education make arbitrary assertions every day. The individuals with whom they deal become unnecessarily angry or guilt-ridden in the absence of any evidence offered for the accusation being made against them. Consider a more detailed case history to help illustrate the crucial application of this point to everyday life.

Case Example of an Arbitrary Assertion

Joe and Melissa have been married for sixteen years. Last year, Joe accepted that he had a gambling addiction. He joined a local chapter of Gamblers Anonymous, a Twelve Steps program for compulsive gamblers.

At first, Melissa was happy Joe sought help. She had suspected that he had a problem for some time and knew that Joe needed help before he was willing to admit it. As time went by, however, Melissa became uneasy. Although she presumed that Joe was not gambling any more, he began to keep his distance. He went to Gamblers Anonymous (G.A.) meetings every night. He began to spend more and more time with G.A. friends, shutting out older friends even if they never gambled.

Melissa started to feel shut out of Joe's life. When she tried to confront him with her feelings, Joe responded: "You are an enabler. For me to have been sick all of these years, you must have been sick too. You made it easier for me to gamble. It doesn't matter if you can't see this. You did it unconsciously. And until you accept that you are diseased, there is no hope for you either."

Melissa became very distressed over Joe's claim. She felt paralyzed and helpless. At other times she felt angry—almost in a rage—but could not even identify what she was angry about. To add insult to injury, Joe revealed one night that he had been relapsing. He admitted to gambling numerous times since beginning his G.A. program.

What disturbed Melissa most about this discovery was that Joe did not seem bothered by it. She learned that his G.A. sponsor—a kind of confidante/therapist who also had a gambling problem—told him not to be "so hard on yourself." It seemed to her that he ought to be at least somewhat hard on himself for gambling when the goal was to quit.

She became confused and started to have anxiety attacks for the first time in her life. She ended up in a therapist's office.

The therapist asked Melissa to invite Joe to a session with her. Joe refused, indicating that Melissa had her own disease and it was good for her to get help, so long as the therapist was a believer in The Twelve Steps.

Melissa could not understand what Joe meant by "diseased." She explained that it was hard enough for her to think of her husband's gambling problem as a disease—a psychological problem, for sure, but not a disease. And the idea that she herself was diseased made her feel like Joe was blaming her for his own problem.

The therapist asked Melissa to try an experiment. She was given the assignment of asking Joe, at an appropriate time when they were alone together at home, if he could explain the reasons *why* he felt she had a disease. Joe seemed irritated at the question and simply replied, "If your therapist is a believer in The Twelve Steps, he should be able to tell you."

But Melissa persisted, and Joe finally told her to read Melody Beattie's book, *Codependent No More*. Melissa did so. While she found the book made some interesting points about not unwittingly encouraging the addict's problem, she still saw no evidence that she herself was diseased, nor an enabler as the author defined the term.

She discussed the issue further with her therapist, who gave her the following task: In the future, whenever Joe made a claim about her (especially with respect to this disease) which she did not understand, she was to calmly respond, "Why?" or "Please explain what you mean."

If Joe refused to answer, or simply became indignant as he had before, she would resolve not to become upset about it. Her therapist predicted that she would find this extremely difficult, and possibly even painful at times, but she needed to learn it as a habit. She needed to learn that nobody, not even her husband, was allowed to make claims without reasons they could explain and defend. While she might not always agree with or necessarily understand her husband, she would at least know that he was making an honest effort when he attempted to provide honest, clearly thought out answers. Nothing less was acceptable.

Discussion of the Case Example

The issue involves much more than mere communication. In the Melissa and Joe example, the issue is cognitive. Joe's cognitive error is in making an arbitrary assertion: he claims that Melissa is diseased and expects her to take this claim on faith.

Melissa's error involves not recognizing Joe's claim as an arbitrary assertion. She first needs to understand what an arbitrary assertion is, and why it has no merit. When Joe (or anyone) makes such assertions in the future, she can learn to put the other individual on the defensive instead of becoming defensive herself.

Once the error of the arbitrary assertion is fully understood, an individual is protected from falling into the trap of believing a mystical therapist. Perhaps common sense ought to be enough to avoid therapists who claim that a client can "transcend" reality and find all the answers with little effort beyond letting the mind go blank. But some mystical therapists are so exploitative that clients will not understand the flaw in the therapeutic technique unless they first understand why arbitrary claims are irrational in the first place.

The client must always be willing to ask the therapist, "Why?" if in doubt about anything. A good therapist wants his point to be understood. He will patiently explain the point as many times as necessary until the client sees it.

A bad therapist wants his arbitrary claims to be accepted on faith. He prefers a client who fails to understand over a client who fails to believe.

Mystical Therapy As Psychological Suicide

Mystical therapy divorces the rational mind from the therapeutic process. Like other forms of bad therapy, it ignores the fact that the reasoning, volitional human mind exists.

Mystical therapy replaces thinking with arbitrary claims about "alternative" levels of reality where facts can be wished away. To the mystic all that matters is that the client willfully suspend consciousness as a route to either improved psychological health or self-understanding. The mystic fails to recognize that thoughts precede emotions and only through the use of the active, reasoning mind will psychological problems gradually resolve themselves.

The mystical approach is akin to seeing a physician for a sprained ankle and having the physician break the ankle rather than treat it. Just as a physician ought to be expected to heal the client's body, a psychotherapist ought to be expected to help the client better utilize the capacity to think and reason. A psychotherapist is, after all, a "doctor" of the mind, and reason represents the tool the human must use to survive, cope and find happiness in life.

Unfortunately, the mystical therapist shows no recognition that a rational faculty even exists, except when ordering the client to shut it off. The overriding goal of any mystical therapist—whether he takes the client to Heaven, Nirvana, a previous lifetime, the Collective Unconscious or the Transcendent Self—is to convince the client to stop thinking.

Mystical therapy, unlike other forms of bad psychotherapy, has no redeeming qualities when practiced consistently. It flunks the test for all seven of my criteria for good psychotherapy. Mystical therapy is almost always devoid of feedback. Who needs feedback if one's logical mind is suspended, anyway? Such therapy is by nature *dis*empowering because it encourages the individual to let go of the very things he needs for both survival and psychological growth: conscious, rational thought and independence.

The client of mystical therapy learns to focus solely on his feelings rather than on reality as the actual *goal* of therapy. Mystical therapy is not problem-focused; it encourages the client to develop new problems (e.g., inventing unresolved conflicts from a former life) rather than try to resolve the problems which inhibit happiness in *this* life.

Mystical therapy adopts neither a systems perspective nor any perspective, for that matter; the attempt to escape from reality, similar to that of the drug abuser, represents a child-like attempt to enjoy the fruits of conscious thought and activity without any of the attendant responsibilities.

Mystical therapy does not constitute a therapeutic alliance because the concept "alliance" implies a rational agreement between two individuals about what should occur as a result of psychotherapy. Mystical therapy, in contrast, involves only the unspoken agreement that running from reality will somehow give the client the simple answer she wants (e.g., to the psychic, "Will I be married by age thirty or not?")

Finally, mystical therapy does not result in an integration of past and present, but rather in a disintegration of consciousness caused by a refusal to think logically about one's problems and emotions.

Mystical therapy prides itself on being "tolerant." And given the outrageous, unscientific claims made by mystical therapists, they certainly have a vested interest in a policy of toleration for toleration's sake.

If no objective standards exist for evaluating what is right or wrong, then sooner or later everything must be accepted—even murder and self-destruction. No relationship, no family, no profession, and no world can survive for long if arbitrary claims are to be accepted as objective fact.

To avoid the hazards of mystical therapy, the therapy consumer needs more than simple common sense. The prospective client must understand the nature of arbitrary claims and why accepting them inevitably leads to a sense of frustration, hopelessness and powerlessness.

Why Psychotherapy Is Not a Right

10

One purpose of this book is to identify the wider impact of psychotherapy on American society, especially over the last several decades when therapy has become more influential. Just as so many people have mistaken or unclear ideas about psychotherapy and what it can and cannot do to help them, many have likewise fallen into the trap of thinking that mental health care is, or at least ought to be, a political and moral right paid for by the government (meaning: everybody else who works).

Numerous mental health associations are usually at the forefront of any attempt to nationalize medical and mental health care. Since so many people have severe emotional problems, they rationalize, then guaranteed psychotherapy or substance abuse treatment "on demand" will alleviate social problems of divorce, crime, drug abuse, and so forth. On this important issue, I take exception to the views of my colleagues in the mental health care establishment.

Many people who think, like myself, that good therapy is possible also leap to the conclusion that good therapy ought to be established as a moral, political right. Others believe that the existence of so much bad therapy requires intensive government intervention and regulation to somehow make the problem go away.

In order to provide an alternative to these conventional views, I will describe the moral and practical arguments *against* any form of government intervention in the fields of medicine and mental health, outside of fraud and objective malpractice.

Why Nobody Has a *Moral* Right
to Mental Health Treatment

Although proponents of the most recent attempt to mandate national health insurance failed to persuade a majority of Americans,[87] the debate over whether people have a *moral* right to health care (including mental health care) remains far from resolved.

The notion that health care is a moral right requires vigorous challenge. Politicians like to claim that the so-called "national interest" must supersede "narrow" interests and that medical/mental health treatment must be guaranteed under the law.

Think carefully about this argument. Is it really in the national interest to alienate health care providers from their patients and clients? Can the emerging managed care bureaucracy, one that many health care providers and patients/clients already resent, be improved by a complex, often arbitrary web of government regulations and directives designed to institutionalize such a system? Can a National Health Board of six or eight politicians actually succeed where free market mechanisms have supposedly failed?

Many are tempted to think that national health insurance, especially a single-payer plan such as the Canadian system, will solve the problem of medical inflation. With the stroke of a politician's pen, it is reasoned, the American system could be streamlined and run like a well-oiled engine thereafter. Each American would have all the health care he desires merely by being born into or acquiring American citizenship. Insurance paperwork would decrease, physicians could regain their professional integrity and, best of all, the kind and compassionate federal (or state) government would remove what is widely viewed as the stench of the profit motive from the medical profession forever.

Think again.

Before examining the impracticality of such a system, one must consider a more fundamental point. Is health care really a moral *right?* "Why, yes," one might reply. "National health insurance means everybody gets the medical care he deserves. Because medical care is a life or death issue, medical treatment has to be viewed as a moral right. The government is obliged to provide its citizens with that right."

What exactly is a "right?" The morality implied by the American Constitution, although never explicitly stated, is that rights are inherent to man's nature. The government cannot "create" or "take away" man's rights—only protect them or fail to protect them. As the philosopher Aristotle pointed out several thousand years ago, man is a rational animal and cannot survive on mere instinct or biological preprogramming as do lower animals. How does man survive? By the use of reason, or, put another way, the free and *uncoerced* use of his individual and independent judgment. I stress the term "uncoerced" because individuals are no longer free to think or reason the moment that force, or even the mere threat of force, is introduced. No mind can think under force or the threat of force; an individual can initiate thought only if actively and voluntarily choosing to do so.

Individual rights, then, protect the freedom of an individual to use his method of survival without the threat of force or coercion from others. Rights apply strictly to freedom of *action;* there is no "right" to the *consequences* of someone else's action. You and I have a right to make bread or to trade with the local baker for bread; but neither you nor I have a right to take the baker's bread (nor even the crust from his bread) without his voluntary, uncoerced consent. If we did possess such a "right," this would mean that the baker is our slave. The same is true of any commodity or service that an individual creates through his own physical and mental efforts.[88]

If this argument sounds too idealistic, one should consider the utter practicality of freedom and individual rights if acted on consistently. In a free society (not to be mistaken for today's highly complex mixture of welfare socialism and free enterprise), all individuals are left free to develop their potential and then benefit through the voluntary exchange of the products of their efforts. A vicious myth persists that nineteenth century capitalism was an era of "robber barons" and cruel indifference. History clearly shows that the Industrial Revolution raised the standard of living for everyone, providing even the *poor* with a lifestyle that would have been the envy of royal monarchs two centuries earlier.[89] There is nothing mean-spirited about an economic system which respects the moral dignity and freedom of individuals and simultaneously allows for unprecedented practical improvements in the standard and quality of human life.

No government can or ever will be able to create the kinds of technological and medical discoveries that Americans increasingly take for granted. Governments fulfill the role, quite appropriately, of the jailers, the police officers and the upholders of private contracts; *force,* not creativity and ingenuity, is by the very nature of government the only arena in which it can excel. Governments can, in mixed welfare-market economies such as the United States, seize, "manage" or redistribute the products of man's efforts, but only *after* the products or technologies are discovered and mass produced by willing, productive individuals.

Most "liberal" and "conservative" politicians understand this fact, which is why so few of them are ideologically committed to socialism. They realize that productive individuals must be left *free enough* to produce a sizable tax base so that the enterprise of government may continue at the involuntary expense of those who provide the wealth in the first place. Today's cynical, often shamelessly hypocritical politicians represent the logical outcome of an economy based upon a perverse mixture of freedom and socialistic redistribution for the so-called public interest.

Whether or not the government ultimately succeeds in its never-ending efforts to nationalize the private practice of medicine, one fact can never be wished away: only uncoerced and reasoning individuals, working in the spirit of *voluntary* and rational cooperation, can create the products and knowledge required for human survival and, in wealthier societies, the luxuries required for the good life. This fact explains why the protection of the individual rights is of paramount importance and why a free society needs a form of strictly *limited* government. A free society requires a government to protect the rights of individuals to create, keep and dispose of the fruits of their efforts as they see fit. A right is violated only through the initiation of force, the threat of force, or objectively provable fraud or deceit.

A police force, a voluntary military and a civil and criminal court system are all necessary in order to avoid the chaos that would inevitably result in the absence of a government monopoly on the use of force. At the same time, strict limits must be placed on the government itself to prevent envious or other opportunistic individuals from seizing the reins of power and imposing force on peaceful citizens, as twentieth century politicians have routinely accomplished in varying degrees. Today's breakdown in social harmony brought about by too much or too little government is exactly what the original American concept of limited government, practiced consistently, was designed to prevent.

Altruistic arguments about compassion, fairness and equity do not work here. One individual's need is not a mortgage on another's life. I am not morally guilty if I earn a million dollars and my neighbor does not. Nor do I have a right to even one penny of his million dollars if he earns it and I do not. The free individual decides who, if anyone, is worthy of his charity; the government has no right to seize part of his income by force and redistribute it to another who allegedly needs it more. Nor does the government have a moral right to take over an entire profession, outlaw private and voluntary contracts between doctors and patients and then determine, by some incomprehensible bureaucratic formula, what constitutes "reasonable" prices.[90]

In the most recent debate over national health insurance, both sides (liberal *and* conservative) took it for granted that the physical and mental effort of health care providers is a national resource to be divided up as any National Health Board or Task Force who manages to seize power sees fit. The debate was strictly limited to the rights of the uninsured, the rights of employers, and the rights of patients. It is a rationalization of unthinkable proportions to presume that a health care provider's practice, creative energies, and rights can be placed on the auction block of Congress and sold to the highest bidder. It is a still greater travesty when health care providers, the very victims whose lives and energies are continuously negotiated away by frantic and confused politicians, endorse such efforts in the name of professional self-interest.

Health care providers confused by the recent explosion of managed care and health maintenance organizations

(HMOs) are the greatest victims of government intervention in the medical profession. They often do not understand that the government regulation they welcome, as the supposed savior of their professional integrity and financial livelihoods, is the very monster that created medical inflation and physician-patient alienation in the first place. The evidence of the past fifty years suggests that the *real* causes of medical inflation include the following: (1) unfair and irrational tax codes (instituted in 1942) which effectively prevent individuals from purchasing health insurance on their own and without reliance on their employers; (2) a thirty year spending spree by both doctors and patients under Medicare and Medicaid programs which pick up the tab for many hospitalizations or, when the government deficit explodes, force private hospitals to cover the losses; and (3) senseless licensing laws that grant physicians a monopoly on certain medical treatments that could just as competently, and far less expensively, be performed by other medical professionals, such as nurses and physician's assistants.[91]

Such factors are further complicated by the fact that insurance companies, operating with full government encouragement and (in some cases) actual subsidies, have adopted the policies of government agencies by managing and, some would argue, actually rationing medical and mental health care. Insurance companies, in my opinion, should not be condemned for merely trying to survive and make a profit in today's overregulated medical marketplace so long as they are honest and do not demand government subsidies to keep them in business. At the same time the indirect creation of such a system by government policies obscures the fact that a genuinely free market has not existed in the field of medicine, including mental health, for at least half a century.

The argument against national health insurance is not a "conservative" one. As any health care provider knows, there is precious little worth conserving in today's government-mandated third-party reimbursement system. Detailed and practical information on free market approaches, designed to *gradually* phase in a free market in the fields of medicine and mental health, are increasingly available to any individual who relies upon introspection instead of anxiety-driven, range-of-the-moment methods of thinking.

At the same time, one should not consider practical free market solutions until first understanding the *morality* of freedom and individual rights as opposed to rule by government force of any kind. Only then will one see that the establishment of a free market in medicine is consistent with both the national interest and the "narrow" interest, as politicians so casually refer to the private practices and skills of health professionals.

Why Universal Mental Health Coverage Is Impossible to Achieve

Since 1965, government intervention in medicine has prevented the marketplace from operating as it normally would. Medicare and Medicaid destroyed the incentive for doctors and patients to spend wisely simply because the government was (and still is) picking up the tab. As Medicare costs exploded, the government began to force hospitals to treat more and more patients at lower and lower prices. In order to avoid bankruptcy, hospitals had no choice except to charge non-Medicare patients more. As a result private insurance companies, who cover non-Medicare patients, had to raise their premiums. So, do not blame the relatively high cost of health insurance on the marketplace.

Blame it on government interference in the marketplace. Today's high premiums did not exist before 1965.

"Universal coverage" cannot simply be *wished* into existence with the stroke of a politician's pen. The Medicare experience should have taught us that *as cost goes down, demand goes up.* Under national health insurance, short-term costs might go down (or at least be hidden in the form of taxes and job losses brought about by employer mandates), but the long-term costs would be devastating to the quality of medical care we now take for granted. Why should this economic principle matter to the average patient? Read on.

Long-Term Consequence #1: Waiting lines are the inevitable outcome of government controlled (or "managed") medicine. Supply cannot possibly keep up with demand, which simply means that providers would not be able to see patients as quickly or as thoroughly. Nor would they have any more incentive than the government-monopolized post office to make sure treatment is efficient and effective.

Canadians already have national health insurance. A colleague of mine, a physician in Canada, reports that the waiting list for a psychiatrist is *twelve to fifteen months.* According to other sources, Canadians also wait eight months for a mammogram; nine months for prostate surgery; and two years for hip replacement surgery. In January 1989, 40 Canadian children were denied heart surgery due to waits. Twenty-four people died in Canada in 1989 while waiting for heart surgery.

The reports from Great Britain's National Health Service (NHS) are no less horrifying. Consider only a few examples.[92]

> In July 1994, England's Health Service Ombudsman announced that his office had received a record 1,384 registered complaints, a 13 percent increase over the previous year.

While complaints to the NHS have grown steadily since 1988, the number investigated has remained the same.

One elderly British man waited four months in a hospital for cancer tests. He was sent home, where he lived alone, on a national holiday. After kidney failure, he was readmitted and then wheeled through the streets in the rain on the way to another hospital.

A British heart attack victim was discharged from the hospital and told to return for a cardiac ultrasound exam. Because he accidentally was put on the "routine" rather than the "soon" list, he had to wait five months for this procedure. Eventually, he was offered surgery, but died after a two-month wait because, once again, he had been placed on the wrong list.

Are these examples of "compassion" and "fairness" as advocates of national health insurance insist? Is there any reason to think that national health insurance would work any different in the United States than it has in Canada and Britain?

Long-Term Consequence #2: Government control of medicine inevitably leads to irrational regulations and moratoriums. In Canada, for example, a political official recently decided that there were too many Cesarean sections performed and that the government would "ensure" that this was reduced by 30 percent over a specified period.[93] Doctors, who are trained to use their independent medical judgment in such matters, are given an impossible choice in socialized systems: either sacrifice their own integrity and the welfare of their patients *or* risk losing their careers if they are caught violating a government ration policy. These sorts of dilemmas represent the future of medicine in America if government intervention continues to expand, regardless of which political party holds power.

Long-Term Consequence #3: Once treatment is established as a legal "right," hypochondriacs and moochers will have a field day. Imagine a group of individuals who go out for lunch every week. Instead of each diner paying his own portion of the bill every time, they mutually agree to split the bill into *equal* parts at every meal. Now suppose that one of these diners is a moocher. Will he really feel any guilt about ordering lobster tail and two desserts since the cost is the same every time? Will he really use any more restraint when his medical treatment is paid for by others as a matter of right? And what about the majority of the group who are not moochers? Will they feel any guilt about ordering more once they see the moocher doing the same? What will happen to the bill once everyone starts ordering without respect to price consideration?

One of my clients graphically illustrated this point when he said: "I may lose my job because of my drug and alcohol abuse. If I lose my job, I will lose my health insurance. But, then again, under national health insurance my medical care will be free. So why should I stop drinking?"

The nonproductive have the greatest reason to celebrate when health care is mandated as a right.

Long-Term Consequence #4: As demand goes up, the government must institute price controls and eventually rationing to avoid massive government deficits. Price controls are currently part of Medicare and Medicaid, which consumers and employers feel in the form of high health insurance costs. Price controls have been necessary under every nationalized health care system in the world.

Under price controls, health care providers must work longer hours for the same (or even less) money. Imagine a boss telling an employee to permanently increase his work week for no additional—or even less—pay. Will the employee's work performance—and overall attitude—be affected? How can a health care provider's work perfor- mance—and his concern for the needs of the individual patient—be affected when he is micromanaged by daily political edicts?

Many psychotherapists find it difficult enough to deal with the requirements of insurance companies, who at least have an incentive to make the regulations somewhat rational in order to stay in business. Imagine if all the regulations came from the federal government in Washington, D.C.!

Long-Term Consequence #5: Providers of medical and psy- chiatric treatment lose their competitive edge in socialized health care systems. Since universal coverage eliminates all financial obstacles to treatment, more individuals are inclined to visit a doctor or psychotherapist at the first sign of symptoms. Conse- quently, providers never have to worry about finding patients to stay in business. Under a free market system (with no govern- ment financing whatsoever), privately practicing doctors face the risk of going out of business if they do not provide excel- lent treatment. Under a government-regulated system there is no incentive to do excellent work since a steady flow of patients is guaranteed forever. Government doctors work for the government—not for patients.

The best providers of medical and mental health treat- ment are competitive, independent individuals who want honest, paying patients. They dislike bureaucracy because their main concern is to provide competent medical care.

They prefer to work either in private practice or in a *voluntary* association of independent providers, such as a privately financed group practice. They cannot—and will not—work with government officials breathing down their backs; and one can be sure that the cream-of-the-crop will no longer be attracted to the medical and mental health professions as government intervention and regulation continues to grow.

Long-Term Consequence #6: Government intervention in the medical marketplace seriously jeopardizes the continued development of medical research and technology. Evidence of this fact already exists in the United States, thanks to the presence of the Medicare program since the mid-1960s. Consider, for example, the effect of government-inspired policies on the performance of autopsies since the 1970s.

> In fact, not so long ago autopsies were considered so vital to the practice of U.S. medicine that they were required for hospital accreditation. Hospitals had to examine at least 20 to 25 percent of deaths to safeguard quality care, ensure the continuing education of doctors, and in general advance medical knowledge. But by the early 1970s things were starting to change . . . By that time hospitals were beginning to feel the impact of legislative changes of the mid-1960s, changes pushing them to operate in an increasingly profit-oriented way.[94]

This example serves as a good illustration of why "free" or cheap health care, provided by government programs such as Medicare since the 1960s, have pushed costs so high that less money is available for private hospitals and research centers to find cures for diseases such as AIDS and cancer.

Never mind the terms used. "Socialized medicine," "universal coverage" and "national health insurance" are essentially the same. In all cases everyone is responsible for everyone else's health care; the self-employed individual who works seventy hours a week and the loafer who mooches off his relatives are treated as equals. Politicians, using arbitrary and narrow standards, decide where to build hospitals and where to send doctors. No longer are such factors the consequence of individual, informed decisions made on a daily basis by free doctors and free patients, voting with their independent decisions in the marketplace. Choice and freedom gradually disappear until eventually nobody realizes they ever existed.

Socialism—and socialized medicine—clearly failed in the Communist countries where government medicine was only one part of a totalitarian package unthinkable to most Americans. In Russia nearly a century of government medicine resulted in agony, despair and ultimately total collapse. In Britain socialized medicine is such a dismal failure that the government now seeks to restore at least part of the private marketplace; sadly, the citizens have become so dependent on government medical handouts that they are terrified to eliminate the system altogether. In Canada there is already some discussion of a return to a free-market system, although it will be difficult to wean Canadians off the handouts as well.

Socialism, because it is incompatible with the need for rational human calculation, simply cannot work.[95] Nevertheless, it is difficult to eradicate socialist programs because, like drug addiction, they destroy the virtues of hope, independence and all that is desirable in human nature.

We need *less* government involvement in medicine, not more.

Good economists who understand the principle of supply and demand as well as market economics have their work cut out for them in devising a means of returning medicine to the private sector, where it belongs.

A number of good ideas merit serious consideration. Objective legal standards must be returned to the field of medical malpractice; it is simply too easy to sue physicians, and everyone is hurt by the resulting erosion of the doctor-patient relationship. Insurance companies need to be deregulated. Medicare and Medicaid—two horribly inefficient and expensive socialist programs—should either be phased out or made voluntary for future generations, who would be free to choose a private plan instead. Tax-free medical accounts (like IRAs) can ease the pain of phasing out Medicare and Medicaid by allowing individuals to receive large tax-breaks and buy their own health insurance, just as they presently buy their own car, homeowners and life insurance policies. It might be too late to save much of today's poor from dependence on Medicaid, but the government has a moral obligation *not* to foster such dependence in future generations of young people. Tax-credits can also be expanded to encourage charitable donations.[96]

Sooner or later Americans have to choose one or the other: capitalism or socialism. Like spoiled adolescents demanding all the freedom of adulthood without any of the responsibility, some of us yearn for socialism despite overwhelming evidence it cannot and will never work. It is time to grow up. We need to tell our protective, paternalistic government "nanny" to get out of our way. In government, as in therapy, freedom must be accompanied by the responsibility and the desire to be free. If we lose these basic values, no government program in the world can save us.

Take the advice of a psychotherapist: *do not let your fears cloud your view of reality.* Always remember that the more involved the government gets in medicine (or any other enterprise where it does not belong), the more necessary it becomes for the government to become still more involved, until eventually it either takes over the enterprise or phases out altogether. Passionate opponents of freedom and capitalism, never in short supply in any culture or era, unfairly and inaccurately blame the present health-care crisis on the free-market. In 1994, they lost the most recent debate on national health insurance, but they will rise again because many otherwise reasonable people still mistakenly believe that health care providers and insurance companies, rather than the government, are to blame for health care inflation.

Because the government has controlled the practice of medicine more tightly than perhaps any other profession in the last fifty years, today's medical system more closely resembles socialism than capitalism. Government intervention in medicine has failed. Health care reform *is* still necessary. We must ultimately choose between a single-payer system of the Canadian model, which is fundamentally flawed for the reasons already discussed, or the enactment of free-market and liability reforms. At this stage of the game, only one road or the other may be taken and there is unlikely to be any turning back.

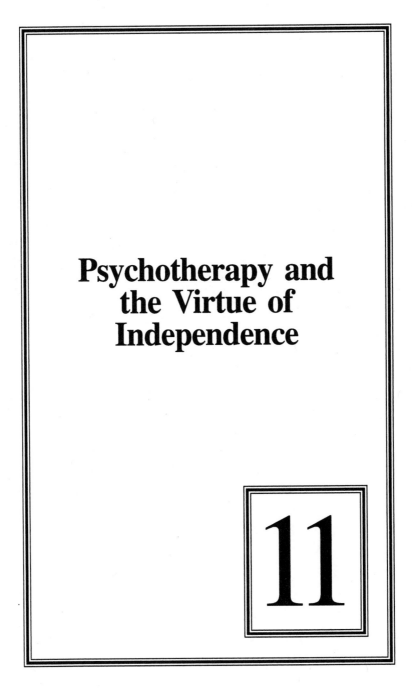

Psychotherapy and the Virtue of Independence

11

Why would any reasonable person, however troubled or vulnerable he might otherwise feel, want to hand over his independence, his common sense, and his unique, individual perspective to one of the many high priests of the psychotherapy profession? What do these people know that he cannot be expected to understand for himself, if guided by the proper principles and assumptions?

Teaching people the proper principles of mental health ought to be the central purpose of psychotherapy. David Seabury suggests that "it is a vital tenet of clinical psychology to *explain principles* rather than to *tell a person what to do*. Wisdom is never dictatorial."[97] Seabury is correct. Therapists can help clients identify their emotions and learn how to better cope with them, but in the end clients must accept responsibility for making their own decisions about their lives.

Relying on the Seabury principle, good therapists tell clients about the capacity for rational introspection and teach them how to use it. The ultimate goal of good psychotherapy is to help people independently use their own minds in the pursuit of psychological achievement and fulfillment. Bad therapy, because of the irrational principles upon which it is based, inevitably leads people to the conclusion that their feelings—and their therapists—are all they have. By eliminating reflective, independent judgment from the process of life, bad therapy makes people dependent on the therapist instead of dependent on themselves.

Rationality, Independence and Psychotherapy

Independence, in the true sense of the word, relies on the understanding that rationality is liberating, not restrictive or repressive. As Nathaniel Branden writes, "If his emotions are to be a source of pleasure to man, not a source of pain, he must learn to *think* about them. Rational awareness is not the 'cold hand' that kills; it is the power that liberates."[98]

The truly independent individual neither rebels for the sake of rebelling (today's permissive trend) nor conforms for the sake of conforming (the old-fashioned, repressive view). The truly independent individual forms convictions rationally, using evidence, and sticks by them unless or until there are good, logical reasons to do otherwise.

Since independence and rationality are intertwined, psychological health depends upon both. Good therapy, therefore, relies upon principles which lead the individual toward independence and rationality rather than away from these virtues.

Psychotherapy—if based upon the proper principles— reinforces (or perhaps even introduces) in an individual the idea that there *are* causes of emotional states over which one does have direct control: ideas and assumptions. It counters the currently popular emphasis on being "psychically liberated" from any and all restrictions on our emotions, even reasonable requirements that we defend our feelings with facts and logic. Without appropriate, self-imposed checks on our emotions, we become more dependent upon others to do our thinking for us. Stanton Peele writes,

> Despite our preoccupation with health and
> with being psychically liberated, we are in-
> creasingly dependent on external agencies
> and less sure of our ability to manage our
> own bodies and our lives.[99]

A basic psychological requirement of an independent mind involves the ability to distinguish between thoughts and emotions. The independent thinker knows his feelings but also wants to trace the origins of the unspoken assumptions which created the feelings in the first place. Even if he requires the help of a psychotherapist, he understands that the purpose of therapy is to help him introspect and discover the causes of his troubling emotions. He is willing to *work* for his mental health.

Dependent minds, on the other hand, are unable to distinguish between thoughts and emotions. Dependent minds know what their feelings are—and little else. Anxiety, sadness and frustration are intolerable to them because they do not know the origin of their feelings, nor do they even understand that feelings have origins. Consequently their lives are reduced to dependence on their biological functions, which is really all that feelings are.

A dependent mind does not understand that basic principles are required to govern even the most mundane aspects of life; he sneers at the idea of principles, dismissing them as rigid, authoritarian, and unsophisticated. Yet his life continues to be plagued by low self-esteem, unexplained anxiety and a pervasive sense of angry helplessness. He pleads with a therapist to "make" his bad feelings go away, and he resents the idea of having to work at it. Moreover, he does not want a therapist to teach him accurate principles about human emotions and introspection. Instead, he wants the therapist to simply tell him what to do.

Independent thinkers are able to handle political and intellectual freedom; in fact, they require it for their very physical and spiritual survival. They can accept nothing on blind faith. They cannot be convinced of an idea until they grasp its basic connection to reality in physical, concrete terms.

A dependent mind, on the other hand, is not only able to live without intellectual and political freedom; he is actually threatened by freedom. Instead of simply having a need for role models and heroes, as even independent thinkers do, he experiences a need to be *ruled.* In politics he expects either a strongman or a benevolent government bureaucrat to handle every aspect of his life—medical care, retirement income, day care, parental leave, disability insurance, and so on. In psychotherapy, he expects a therapist who will "make" him feel better than a therapist who will teach him the principles and the skills necessary for a happier, healthier life.

The dependent mind and the bad therapist are a perfect match for one another. The dependent individual wants to be dictated to; the bad therapist needs to dictate.

It does not matter if the individual is encouraged to surrender his responsibility—and his freedom—to his Freudian unconscious, to his mysterious Higher Power, to the conditioning stimulus or to the therapist himself. The central point is that bad therapy *disempowers* an individual by teaching him that the mind and the body—his thoughts and emotions—are at war with each other; he is not allowed to see that mind and body, conscious and subconscious, can be successfully integrated with time and effort. Only good therapy—or, more fundamentally, a rational philosophy of life—can lead an individual to understand the basic integration of thoughts and emotions required for a psychologically healthy existence.

Independence is not the same as intelligence. Many intelligent people are highly dependent. In fact, bad therapists and other contemporary intellectuals are often quite dependent individuals, even though they may mask it under a facade of pseudo-self-esteem or even arrogance.

Consider, for example, the experienced psychotherapist who approaches his colleague and complains, "I don't know what to do with these panic-stricken people who come into my office. They feel that their world is collapsing, and who am *I* to tell them otherwise?"

Most of this therapist's clients would be horrified to know he made such a statement; yet, given his lack of a rational perspective on emotions, how can one find fault with his logic? Who could expect him to think otherwise after years of being assaulted with Freudian, behaviorist, mystical and anti-male ideas?

Or, consider the case of the client who was going through an extremely bitter divorce and needed a child custody evaluation for court. The man and his estranged wife together attended a session with a respected psychotherapist appointed to make, in essence, the ultimate decision about custody upon which the judge could be expected to rely. The man later commented that the therapist looked as if she were about to burst into tears during the session. Apparently she felt the couple's pain and anger so intensely that she was unable to be of much help. Yet what else can one expect from therapists taught that empathy, not judgment, is the single most important skill of a psychotherapist?

Conversely, many uneducated individuals are quite independent and self-reliant in their psychological outlooks, even if they do not have a great deal of knowledge about psychological theories. Through my own experience in practicing psychotherapy, I can verify that many helpful techniques, ideas and suggestions have come from clients themselves. Clients teach me a great deal. At the same time, I can count on one hand the number of therapists who have taught me anything worthwhile. This is not necessarily an attack on the intelligence or intentions of therapists I have encountered. It is, however, an attack on the quality of the theoretical principles and philosophies most therapists bring to their practices.

Independent yet uneducated individuals tend to give authority figures, such as intellectuals and psychotherapists, the benefit of the doubt. I have repeatedly observed, sadly, that when therapists rely on mistaken philosophies, they tend to resort to subtle intimidation to get clients to accept theories which have no basis in reality. I cannot count the number of referred clients I have received who were emotionally damaged, intentionally or otherwise, by their previous therapists. Here are a mere handful of examples:

> "My therapist told me I'm in denial just because I have a glass of wine at dinner every other night! Am I really an alcoholic?"

> "The therapist told me I'm not ready for therapy—what does this mean? Does this mean I'm a hopeless case?"

> "The therapist told me I was trying to terminate prematurely. What does this mean? I cut off the therapy because it wasn't helping. The therapist actually called me at home and told me that I am not a very thoughtful person to treat her like this."

> "I took my daughter to family counseling and the therapist put words in her mouth. The therapist said to her, 'You're angry, aren't you, Melissa?' and Melissa claimed that she was. Yet Melissa has never said or done anything to suggest this is the case."

A fair portion of my own practice has been spent undoing the damage to the self-esteem of conscientious, otherwise independent individuals by therapists with mistaken ideas.

The Impact of Bad Therapy on Society

In contemporary America bad therapists have accomplished their primary goal. We are now a society of feelers. Everyone has a right to his feelings—not simply to feel them but to have them accepted as truths. We no longer repress our emotions, and it amounts to educational heresy to introduce the concept of reason into university humanities departments, much less first grade.

As a culture we are supposedly more "humanistic." We are supposedly more "humanitarian," more "compassionate," more "supportive" and "caring" and "non-judgmental" in our approach with one another. Yet how do we explain the fact that—in everyday life—we are becoming less courteous toward one another? That we sue each other more, that we say "excuse me" less often and that acts of *voluntary* kindness are rarer? And how do we explain the unprecedented degree of violence? And drug abuse? And the general attitude of cynicism and helplessness which pervades our once optimistic and hopeful society?

The answer is clear to a rational therapist because the principles that apply on the individual level apply equally on the social level. Under the influence of bad therapy and deterministic philosophy, our widely recognized social, economic and spiritual deterioration continues unabated. No other outcome is possible if feelings—and feelings alone—are used to guide one's actions and decisions.

Under the dominance of the emotionalist perspective, especially over the last three decades, placing one's feelings above all else has become the norm. But feelings without reference to reality are no less destructive than reality without reference to feelings. In other words, "do-as-you-feel" subjectivism has been no more successful than "do-as-I-say" dogmatism. It is only through establishing harmony between feelings and reality, with the help of reason and introspection, that psychological health can be achieved and maintained.

Introspection places responsibility for assessing the truth or falsehood of a situation in individual hands—but demands that each individual use objective, rational standards. When more individuals practice introspection and more therapists utilize good cognitive methods, we can expect society to be a better place to live.

It is critical that psychotherapists—who, perhaps more than other professionals, have the greatest influence on *individual* lives—play a major role in reintroducing logic and reason into the lives of troubled people. Cognitive therapy, introspection and teaching a rational philosophy of life can all contribute to a society in which there is less crime, less drug addiction and less dependence on external authorities for running every aspect of our lives. Most importantly, cognitive principles can lead more individuals to be happy.

A healthy society starts with psychologically healthy individuals who have high self-esteem and are independent. Such virtues are by-products of rationality.

Rationality includes a recognition that feelings are not the same as facts, and that consequently a process of reason—including introspection—needs to be developed as a daily habit from the earliest age possible.

The *ideas* upon which bad therapy relies—and which many otherwise decent, intelligent psychotherapists and clients have allowed themselves to accept—are the root cause of many of today's social problems. The cure for the unhappy society is the same as the cure for the unhappy individual: the correction of mistaken, illogical assumptions.

The method is good therapy.

Appendix

Case Examples of Introspection Method

Feeling: "My teenage son does not love me. I slave for him, day and night. He does not appreciate all I do for him. Here I have provided him with the best education, the best clothes, and almost everything he could ask for. What is wrong with him? Why does he not love me? I must have done something wrong as a parent."

Facts Which Support This Conclusion:

1. My son's behaviors are clearly not loving, especially lately. He ignores me when I come home at the end of the day. He generally leaves a room as soon as I enter, without acknowledging me. He does not show me any physical affection, such as hugging, as he used to do when he was younger.
2. I overheard my son telling his friend on the telephone that he can't wait to grow up and get away from me.
3. He does not tell me where he's going and when he'll be home unless nagged or coerced into doing so. He has never been so secretive in the past.
4. He mocks my political beliefs, my religious beliefs, my moral values, and just about everything I think is true.

Facts Which Support a Different Conclusion:

1. I have done everything in my power and knowl-
    edge to be a good parent. I have made mistakes,
    but I have also learned from them and applied
    the new knowledge as the opportunity arose. I
    always apologize when I do something that I
    later see as wrong or irrational.
2. I can think of no actions on my part that would
    lead him to act in this way. I act and think just
    like I always have.
3. My experiences with my older child and other
    parents' experiences suggest that the teenage
    years are a time when a child likes and needs to
    become more independent. I must respect this
    fact if I am to get anywhere with him.
4. I choose to "slave" for him. He has not been
    asking me to do all of these things, and in some
    cases, such as picking out his clothes, he might
    not even want me to do these things for him. I
    may be turning myself into a self-sacrificial
    "martyr" and maybe this gets on his nerves.

*Based on the above, do I have sufficient data to support my
emotional conclusion?*

It doesn't seem that way. First of all, I am not a bad
parent. I can only be a bad parent if I fail to raise
my son in the best way I know how and if I fail to
be thorough and conscientious about it. Would I be
having this conversation with myself right now if I
were not thorough and conscientious? I cannot say
that I'm a bad parent simply for not being able to
read my son's mind.

Furthermore, before I conclude that my son does not love me, I need to rule out a number of other hypotheses. First of all, I need to make sure I am not being a martyr. Another possible hypothesis is that he is trying to become more independent, as many kids are known to do at this age. Finally, I need to remember that it is not his job to make me happy. He is becoming a young adult, and it is his role actually to become more self-absorbed and less concerned with pleasing his parents. Within reasonable limits, this is probably a healthy and even necessary stage of his development.

Rational Course(s) of Action/Methods for "Letting Go" of Irrational Conclusion:

1. I need to be up front with him about the martyr issue and ask him if I am doing too much for him, such as buying him clothes when maybe he wants more independence in such decisions. If he is defensive and will not cooperate with this discussion, then I can simply try experiments. For example, I can just stop picking out his clothes for him and see if he reacts negatively.

2. I need to consider the possibility his behavior is largely healthy and keep in mind that many teenagers, including my older child, did the same thing. While this fact does not necessarily justify his rudeness toward me, it might at least explain some of his behavior and help me to allow him a little "emotional room" without, of course, endorsing behaviors that I see as harmful to himself or others.

3. Keeping the above in mind, let him know that his behaviors sometimes hurt my feelings and, while I understand he has a right to his own life, I have rights as well.

4. Turn this into a positive [psychological entrepreneurism]—try to think of this as a time of increased independence for myself. My son does not need me emotionally like he used to. This frees me up to put my emotional energy into other areas such as my friendships and my marital relationship. Maybe my husband and I can actually consider going to the beach for a weekend without any kids, for the first time in years.

Feeling: "I want a drink. But I am powerless over alcohol. There is no cause of my desire to drink except perhaps a genetic one. It just happens. I must immediately go to my AA group so that they can keep me from drinking. I would be helpless without them."

Facts Which Support This Conclusion:

1. The urge to drink is a compulsion, and a very strong one.

2. A support group, such as AA, can be a critical part of stopping one's drinking.

3. Since in the past I usually gave in to the urge to drink, it is quite natural to think that I am powerless over alcohol.

4. I am very lonely right now and the AA group naturally takes on added importance since I have decided to back away from my alcohol and drug-abusing friends.

Facts Which Support a Different Conclusion:

1. All feelings have causes, including the feeling that I want a drink. Feelings are consequences of thoughts and assumptions. The thought that ran through my head, at the very moment I craved the drink, was this: "I failed today at work. I need to console myself with a drink to forget about it."

2. Many people stop compulsive drinking, even without AA and other support groups. I know that it is at least possible for some people to stop without such a group.

3. At present, I have provided myself with no incentives to stop drinking. I have not yet developed any hobbies or friendships which are not self-destructive. It seems possible that if I had such nondestructive values in my life, the incentive would be greater not to run out and get a drink at the first sign of stress.

4. I chose not to drink last Thursday when the compulsion was just as strong if not stronger. I did it without going to a meeting since there was no meeting to attend at the time. By the next day the urge to drink was completely gone and I made it to work on time.

Based on the above, do I have sufficient data to support my emotional conclusion?

No. Numerous other hypotheses are possible. First of all, I need to consider the fact that my thoughts, and not some external process, are creating my urge to drink. I can change my thoughts or, at the very

least, make a resolution not to act on particular thoughts.
Last Thursday offers strong evidence in support of this
theory. I chose not to drink that day, and I did not even
need to go to an AA meeting. If I can do this once, it
is certainly possible, if not easy at first, to do this many
times. A second hypothesis has to do with the kind of
rational values I have in my life. Because drinking has
always been my chief value, and I have not yet replaced it with anything even though I have stopped it,
I need to consider that the urge to drink will be further
reduced as I bring other interests and values into my
life. I need to keep in mind that many people have
stopped drinking without the help of AA. While this
does not necessarily mean that I should quit AA tomorrow, it should give me hope that I need not rely on
others to stop my drinking for me.

*Rational Course(s) of Action/Methods for "Letting Go" of
Irrational Conclusion:*

1. Pursue therapy with a professional who can help
    me change my negative thinking habits and re-
    inforce the idea that I have choices and do not
    have to depend solely on a Higher Power or
    group to keep me from drinking.
2. Spend at least thirty minutes every single day de-
    veloping a more rational value system. Engage
    myself in activities that are not self-destructive.
    Don't worry too much about whether or not I enjoy
    them because at first I will probably not enjoy
    anything that is not self-destructive. This feeling is
    actually quite normal because I have engaged in
    destructive behaviors for so long that I no longer
    feel the possibility of living any other way.

3. Turn this negative experience into a positive [psychological entrepreneurism]. Treat it as an opportunity to develop interests and achieve goals I long ago placed aside. Ask myself each day what new opportunity is opened up by the end of my drinking days.

4. Try not to become addicted to a Twelve Steps program. Appreciate the group for what it has to offer me but do not let it stand in the way of achieving other goals and developing other interests. For every hour I spend at a meeting, I need to make a strong commitment to myself that I will spend an additional hour developing a healthy interest or goal outside of the group. I need to keep track of these hours rigidly in order for this technique to work. Do not let anyone stand in the way of this.

Feeling: "My wife and I have not had sex in several months. This means our relationship is in trouble. She does not love me and I must be performing poorly as a man."

Facts Which Support This Conclusion:

1. Sex is a central component of a healthy romantic relationship. It is valid to feel concern if a partner stops showing interest in it.

2. Because sex is a delicate subject, my wife might indeed be dissatisfied in some way and feels unable to tell me.

3. Women, in particular, might find it difficult to go ahead with sexual intercourse if something is bothering them. Her apparent lack of interest

could indeed be a warning signal that something is wrong.

Facts Which Support a Different Conclusion:

1. Although we have not had sex in several months, we do hold and touch each other every night and she clearly seems to enjoy this.
2. She has made several trips to the doctor lately and is frustrated that he has been unable, so far, to come up with a clear diagnosis for her occasional headaches and dizzy spells.
3. She recently went back to work full-time and this might be a difficult transition for her. This is the first time she has worked full-time since our two kids were born.

Based on the above, do I have sufficient data to support my emotional conclusion?

No. I first need to rule out several other hypotheses before assuming my worst-case scenario is true. The fact that she enjoys holding and touching clearly flies in the face of the idea that she no longer loves me. I also need to consider the possibility that her medical question might be bothering her, making it difficult for her to let go and enjoy sexual intercourse. Another hypothesis is that she is stressed out about her work and unable to enjoy sex.

Rational Course(s) of Action/Methods for "Letting Go" of Irrational Conclusion:

1. Continue holding and touching at night, and not let my feelings of hurt and anger about lack of

sex get in the way of this goal. After all, we both enjoy holding each other and it's more important than ever right now since we're not having sex.

2. Ask her more detailed questions about her work, and look to see if she has any insecurities or objective stressors on the job that may be making it hard for her to relax. See if I can get her to talk about this; maybe the fact I'm showing some interest will be enough to make her feel better.

3. Use the same approach about the medical problem. Wait until the next appointment with her doctor to see if he determines a diagnosis. Consider going to the doctor with her, both as a way to be supportive and to ensure that I know everything he is telling her.

4. If we're both comfortable, the option always exists to try other forms of sexual expression, outside of sexual intercourse, that may be fulfilling for both of us to get through this period (oral sex and mutual masturbation are two examples).

5. Turn the negative into a positive [psychological entrepreneurism]—without disregarding the fact that this issue ultimately needs resolution, recognize that it might present opportunities to enjoy the relationship in other ways, such as paying more attention to hugging, kissing or other nonsexual yet still physical forms of expression.

6. If none of these approaches work, I can simply talk to my wife directly about this concern. If she becomes defensive or refuses to deal with it, I can remain calm and ask that we address this issue with the help of a third party such as a counselor. I can appeal to her own sense of

self-interest and ask if *she* is really happy leaving this unresolved.

Feeling: "My wife is having an affair. I can just feel it."

Facts Which Support This Conclusion:

1. She is late from work almost every night and never has a reasonable excuse.
2. She has shown no interest in sex for the past six months and shows no interest in any kind of physical contact at all.
3. She told me she was on the phone with her friend Diane, but I could hear that the voice on the other end was that of a man.
4. She does not want to take a vacation this summer as we usually plan to do.
5. In a recent fight she told me that she no longer loves me; she later denied that she feels this way.
6. She receives mail from a man I do not know, and she grabs it from me before I can look at it.
7. She is generally evasive and mysterious, qualities I have never observed in her before now.

Facts Which Support a Different Conclusion:

1. When confronted, she denies that she is having an affair. I have never known her to be a lying person.
2. She continues to act like herself when she is around the house—doing household chores, errands, reading, watching television, and so on.

Based on the above, do I have sufficient data to support my emotional conclusions?

> I do not yet have proof, but I have very strong support for my feeling. All of her behaviors suggest that she has something to hide and that it is likely that her secret is some kind of romantic affair with a man. There are only two facts which seem to support the opposite conclusion. One is that she has never been a lying person, although I know for a fact that she has lied lately. The other is that she acts like herself when she is around the house, except this ignores the fact that she is generally not around the house, and when she is home, she does not give me any more attention than one would a roommate. I need to face the fact that something is going on and that an affair is a very likely hypothesis.

Rational Course(s) of Action:

1. Emotionally disengage from the relationship. Build up an emotional/social support network, if one does not exist already. Face the fact that the marriage might be ending, and although it will be hard for me to accept this right away, I need to start building a new life for myself. I need to renew old acquaintances and friendships and tell people whom I trust about what I think is going on.

2. Assume that my wife will continue to be evasive about the subject. Try once again to confront her and when she denies anything is going on, as is likely, show her the evidence that has

led me to this conclusion. Ask her if there is any evidence I am leaving out which I should be factoring in.

3. Consider seeing a therapist or some kind of professional confidante so that I do not have to handle this ordeal alone. I will find it extremely hard to maintain objectivity during such a difficult period. This situation is like a death, and I will inevitably have all kinds of psychological symptoms. In some respects breakups are even worse than death because the "dying" is happening right before my very eyes and my wife refuses to admit it.

4. Try not to fall into the trap of following my wife around so as to catch her in the act, tempting as this might be. While I might have every moral right to take these steps, it will likely inflict unnecessary extra pain on myself and distract me from my need to disengage emotionally from this marriage. Try to remember that she has always been a good, honest person and for this reason it must be very hard for her to keep lying like this. Keep confronting her with the inconsistencies in her behavior, of which there are many, and trust that sooner or later she has to break. She is not a chronic liar, so she cannot be very good at this dishonest arrangement for long.

5. Try to remember that I am not as powerless as I might feel. Remember that as I make an effort to cope with this situation, I am preparing myself for the future and she, on the other hand, will have a big mess on her hands. What if the man dumps her? Then she will have lost both him and

me. What happens when she realizes how much she is throwing away by pushing me aside? She will have to go through pain, just like I am going through pain now. The difference is that I will already be through most of my pain, and she will be pleading with me for forgiveness. Although I feel out of control now, she is really the one who has placed her life out of control.

6. Try not to blame the man she is presumably sleeping with. Even if he is an evil person, he is not forcing her to see him. She is making her own choices. And for all I know, she might not even have told him that she is married. If I spend my energy on thinking about him, then it will also take away the strength I need to face the fact that my marriage is probably ending.

Feeling: "Tom does not want to marry me. This means he is commitment-phobic, just like the psychologist on t.v. says most men are. I want to give him an ultimatum. Yet I also am afraid he'll call my bluff and say 'OK, it's over.' I am hopelessly confused and frightened. I don't know what to do."

Facts Which Support This Conclusion:

1. Tom is evasive about the subject of marriage, even when I bring it up in a nice way. He gets all stiff and nervous and asks, "Why do we need to rock the boat? Things are just fine as they are."
2. Marriage certainly is a form of commitment, and Tom clearly seems afraid to embark on it.

3. It is a documented fact that some men (and some women) fear commitment for a variety of reasons.

Facts Which Support a Different Conclusion(s):

1. Tom and I have lived together for several years. We are compatible, do loving things for one another, and in almost all respects are no different from a happily married couple.
2. Tom says that he really likes things the way they are, and I see no reason to question this. I have never known him to lie to me. For the most part, I like things the way they are too.
3. Tom was married once before and had a horribly bitter divorce. The divorce dragged on for a year and his ex-wife tried to extract an unreasonable amount of money from his business. He never told me all of the details, but I feel sure it was horribly painful for him.

Based on the above, do I have sufficient data to support my emotional conclusion?

No. I first have to rule out several other hypotheses. First, I have to consider that Tom's fears from his first marriage might be getting in the way. I also need to factor in that we are both very happy with each other before I make the hasty generalization that he no longer loves me. Quite the contrary: he may love me so much that he is terrified, rationally or not, of "messing things up" by getting married. I owe it to myself and to him to rule out these hypotheses before acting on my feelings.

Rational Course(s) of Action/Methods for "Letting Go" of Irrational Conclusion:

1. Whenever I become fearful, reinforce to myself the fact that our lives are really very happy and that being unmarried does not, in and of itself, change this fact.

2. Introspect, with a therapist's help if necessary, and discover the reasons why I want to be married to Tom. Make sure that all of the reasons are logical and determine if some of them are perhaps illogical.

3. Ask Tom to do the same as a compromise. Ask him to look inward, perhaps with the help of a therapist, and determine all of the reasons for not wanting to get married. Try to convince myself, and then him, that his willingness to introspect is perhaps even more important than whether or not we ultimately get married.

4. Ask myself if there are financial or other practical reasons why I am uncomfortable being unmarried since marriage is a legal agreement. Also check into the state laws to determine if a common law marriage exists after a certain number of years living together. Ask Tom to write up a will.

5. If, after introspecting, I discover that I do have some valid reasons for wanting to get married, then work hard not to become defensive with Tom. Remember that the worst way to handle a defensive person is to become defensive in turn. Although I might feel inside that it is cruel and unjust of him not to marry me, I must understand that he is afraid, perhaps more afraid than I am, and that only by discovering the origins of

this fear can we ultimately resolve the problem. As long as I see him as willing to try and resolve the problem, it serves *my* interest not to rush him and just let him see for himself what his fears are.

6. Psychological entrepreneurism: treat this as an opportunity to help Tom develop respect for me. Remember that men need to respect women just as much as women need to respect men. A man often loses respect for a woman if she becomes overemotional and clings to him. It is important that I stay rational, that I hold my ground on an issue which is important to me but at the same time I stay calm and prove that I have the strength to take care of myself with or without him.

Feeling: "I fear my daughter has a drug problem."

Facts Which Support This Conclusion:

1. She stays out past midnight most nights; sometimes she is gone all night and refuses to say where she went.
2. According to my neighbor's son, she is hanging out with kids known to be the drug users in the school.
3. She has become extremely emotional and sullen in the last few months.
4. Her grades have gone from Bs to Cs and Ds in a short period of time.
5. Her clothes smell of marijuana.
6. I found drug paraphernalia in her bedroom.
7. I have caught her in numerous lies; she never used to be a liar.

Facts Which Support A Different Conclusion(s):

1. When confronted, she denies using drugs.
2. A random urine test, done through her physician, came up negative.
3. I have always taught my daughter not to use drugs, and she is well aware of the negative long-term physical and psychological effects of drug use.
4. Although she has dropped most of her wholesome friends, she is still friends with Mary, whom I know for a fact is not a drug user.

Based on the above, do I have sufficient data to support my emotional conclusion?

I do not have eyewitness proof yet, but the evidence strongly suggests my feeling is accurate. The alternative hypotheses are easily eliminated. According to what I've read, drug users are known for lying about their use, so her denial means little by itself. Urine tests, as her physician explained, sometimes cannot detect drugs that have already left her body. If she is able to lie to me, then she is certainly able to lie to her friend Mary and ignore her knowledge about how deadly drugs can be.

Rational Course(s) of Action:

1. Severely restrict her free time alone. Using the freedom/responsibility principle, tell her that she can regain her freedom only when she shows appropriate responsibility. Grades are one way to measure her responsibility.
2. Work closely with her father because she can be expected to struggle and we need to have a strong

and united front. Any differences between him and me must be placed aside. In a war, allied countries set aside their differences and unite in a common, overriding goal. The same principle applies here.

3. Confront her on every detail I find, as I find it, to suggest that she is using drugs. Do not keep anything a secret, because it will only make it easier for her to lie and evade. If I think I smell drugs, tell her. If I notice she's half an hour late, tell her. Be a real pain in the neck, holding her accountable for every tiny detail. Expect to lose any hint of positive relationship with her during this period. If she stays on drugs, I'll lose it anyway.

4. Insist that she agree to more regular, yet still random, urine tests, once again using the freedom/responsibility principle. When she shows more responsibility in her attitudes and behaviors, then she can expect to be left alone.

5. Seek professional help for the likely tensions these strategies will create. Be sure to pick a therapist that shares the beliefs of my husband and me. Do not base the selection of a therapist on my daughter's feelings; if she chooses to stay in a state of denial, then her judgment cannot be trusted anyway. The therapist is really for the parents to help us better cope with our daughter and not let her destroy her life. I hope later on she will open up to the therapist and share some of her own troubles. But the focus right now is to get her off the drugs and hold her accountable for her actions.

6. Although it is hard, try to look at the positives in the midst of the negatives. I have discovered

and, more importantly, faced up to this problem before it's completely out of hand. Something must have been wrong for her to have started using drugs in the first place, especially when she knows better. This period of confrontation, while painful, should be able to help us get to the root of her problems.

Feeling: "My parents messed me up. By not providing me with the emotional support and nurturance I needed as a child, I failed to develop a healthy sense of self-esteem. This fact explains why I have failed in life, and also why I'll never amount to anything. I *hate* my parents."

Facts Which Support This Conclusion:

1. My parents did not, in fact, provide me with the nurturing a child needs to develop a healthy sense of self-esteem. They taught me that I am guilty of "original sin," which means I am guilty by my very nature as a human being—that I am guilty for having been born. They frequently told me that they wished I had never been born so that they could have done something with their lives. They never encouraged me or complimented me for doing well; I only heard criticism when I did poorly, and these criticisms were typically harsh and exaggerated.
2. My parents did not offer to send me to college, although their income was high enough that they could have helped me out. They simply told me I was too stupid to amount to anything.

3. I was laughed at whenever I tried to take some initiative and told by my parents that initiative was futile and a waste of time.

Facts Which Support A Different Conclusion(s):

1. I have evidence to show that my parents were not raised with self-esteem either. In fact, their parents were even worse; they physically abused them as children. I cannot recognize the effect of my childhood on me if I refuse to recognize the effect of their childhoods on their opinions, values and behaviors.

2. I am making a sweeping generalization with respect to having "failed in life." First of all, I am only forty. My life is only half over—or, put more positively, half unlived. I have had many successes in life, especially considering my bad start. I managed to complete two years of college on my own, for example. After one bad marriage I managed to find a spouse whom I love very much and who cares for me in return.

3. I have certainly failed a lot in life. But it is again a hasty generalization to conclude that all of these failures are the direct cause of low self-esteem. For instance, I dropped out of college for several reasons. One was the high cost of tuition, combined with the fact that I did not realize student loans were available from both the government and private banks. I simply did not have the appropriate information; and, in all honesty, I could have made a better effort to investigate financial aid than I did at the time. I also was not really sure what I wanted to pursue as a major; this problem afflicts many students, even those with

relatively high self-esteem. Perhaps it was better to drop out then since I had no idea where I wanted to go with my studies. I also was forced to learn business skills I might not otherwise have learned so early in life.

Based on the above, do I have sufficient data to support my emotional conclusion?

No, I don't think so. My emotional conclusion is that my parents are evil and have determined every choice, every action and every detail of my life up to this point. In reality, it is my subconscious conclusions—such as the idea that I am guilty by virtue of being alive—which have created my problems. It is true that my parents introduced me to these ideas and reinforced them over and over in the early years of my life. Yet they were also introduced to such ideas in their own childhood, and they simply passed them on to me. While I need to hold them responsible for their actions, I also need to temper my harsh judgment of them against the fact that they were every bit as victimized as I was—in fact, more so.

Rational Course(s) of Action/Methods for "Letting Go" of Irrational Conclusion:

1. Consciously work on countering the hasty, emotional generalization that my parents are the cause of all my current problems. Reality is rarely that simple, and as already demonstrated it is not that simple in my case either.
2. Transfer my anger at my parents, as people, to the *ideas* which are the real root of my problems (and their own problems). For example,

examine the absurdity of the idea that an individual is guilty simply for being born (i.e., original sin). I did not choose to be born, and there is no logical reason to feel guilty simply because I am a human being. I cannot take responsibility for anything except my own actions and choices.

3. Make two lists. One list will include all the things it is too late to change about myself (e.g., the fact that I did not finish college at twenty-one). The other list will include all the things which I still *can* change—e.g., I can still finish college and pursue a career in teaching, which I now realize I always wanted to do. My kids are growing up rapidly and money is no longer the issue it once was.

4. Discover the virtue of independent judgment. Learn to judge myself objectively just as I try to judge everything else in life. Realize that my parents did not judge me objectively—they were irrational and simply looked for the negative in me. Much of my low self-esteem is the remnant of this earlier era; some of my subconscious conclusions from childhood (e.g., "I am worthless, since my parents say so") have still not caught up to the reality that I am an adult and free to judge objectively if I wish. I do not have to use the crazy standards my parents used.

5. "Reprogram" myself with the help of a good psychotherapist—a therapist who rejects the idea that individuals are determined by family, society, and other forms of conditioning. Find a therapist who recognizes that I can use my brain to learn to think in a different, accurate way.

Feeling: "I am not a whole person without a man. It is terrible that I am thirty-two and unmarried. Something must be wrong with me. I cannot be complete and normal until I have a man in my life."

Facts Which Support This Conclusion:

1. It is hard to be alone. It is much nicer to sleep with a spouse or lover every night than it is to sleep alone. It is nicer to have one regular sexual partner instead of continually looking for a new one.
2. My life is, in fact, not complete without a spouse or significant other. There is a good reason why men and women who marry live longer. If the match is a good one, their lives are generally happier.
3. Thirty-two is not old but is a bit old to have not yet married, at least by purely statistical standards. Perhaps there are reasons for this which I need to identify. Perhaps some of these reasons are under my control, and some of them are not.

Facts Which Support A Different Conclusion(s):

1. I am a whole, unique individual person whether I am married or not. My marital status does not, by itself, say anything about my worth or competence as an individual.
2. Being thirty-two and unmarried could mean that I have been conscientiously seeking an appropriate partner—rather than "settling" as so many others do—and simply have not found that individual yet.

3. My marital status says nothing whatsoever about my worth and competencies in other areas of life—e.g., career, social life, personal friendships, extracurricular activities. In fact, these other activities say much more about my competence than does the simple fact of being married or unmarried.

Based on the above, do I have sufficient data to support my emotional conclusion?

No. While my dissatisfaction for being single stems from a normal need which virtually all human beings have—for romantic involvement with someone—there is no basis for allowing my self-worth to depend on it. And many explanations are possible for my still being unmarried. It would be arbitrary to conclude that I am worthless simply because I am not yet married. In fact, just the opposite could be true. It seems more likely that I'm not married because I have been quite conscientious and discriminating in my choice of partners and because I have worked really hard to get my career to where it currently is. Perhaps I wasn't ready to marry before. I need to stop confusing loneliness with worthlessness.

Rational Course(s) of Action/Methods for "Letting Go" of Irrational Conclusion:

1. Challenge my idea of marriage. Many people— many women in particular—are raised with the false idea that a marriage consists of two "halves," almost as if each person gave up "half" of himself in order to join in a union. Tradition-

ally, men gave up their rational "half" to cater to the emotional whims of his wife; and women gave up their rational "half" to stay home with the kids and play the role of permanent house-wife (as opposed to the first few years of the child's life), even if this was not a role that suited them. In reality, a healthy marriage consists of two complete, integrated individuals: two individuals with long-term goals and the emotional skills required to live life to the fullest.

2. Once convinced of this idea logically, then reinforce it whenever possible to counter the subconscious conclusion that marriage is just the reverse. Tell myself to be patient; such a socially prevalent conclusion can take time to change but *will* change with consistent, conscientious effort.

3. In the area of dating, develop a time budget. Make sure that I treat my time with the same respect as my money and other possessions. I would not let anyone steal my money; do not let anyone steal my time, either. Do not go out on a second date with a man I know that I can never be attracted to, simply to avoid hurting his feelings. I am not sparing his feelings; I am only misleading him and postponing the day that I inevitably turn him down. More important, the evening I spent with him might have been the evening I met the man who is an appropriate match for me. Life is too short, and too valuable, to waste time.

4. Adopt the approach of a psychological entrepreneur. Identify the positive aspects of being single and remind myself of them: for instance, having complete control over my own social schedule

without having to consider the opinion of a mate. Take the attitude that, "If I am still single, there must be good reasons for it. Perhaps, subconsciously, I am not convinced I am ready for a committed relationship. I ought to examine my feelings about commitment very closely. If they are based on mistaken assumptions or on facts which no longer apply to me, then I need to change my way of thinking. Otherwise I will shy away from potentially good partners out of a fear of becoming committed." A good therapist can help get this process of introspection moving.

Feeling: "I don't want to think my way out of my problems. Besides, being rational means taking a Pollyanna-ish, simplistic view of life. Life is not that simple. Feelings can be very complicated; life can be very complicated. I resent the idea that my feelings must be ignored in the name of 'rationality.' "

Facts Which Support This Conclusion:

1. Sometimes people who want to be rational do take an over-simplistic view of life.
2. Many people who claim to be "rational" are really individuals who ignore or repress their feelings, and deep down believe that feelings are bad.
3. Feelings can certainly be complicated, and often are the cause of great pain and suffering.
4. Life can also be quite complicated.

Facts Which Support A Different Conclusion(s):

1. Being rational does not mean ignoring or repressing one's feeling. Being rational simply

means not using one's feelings as the exclusive or primary method for discovering the truth of what is happening in reality.

2. Being rational means a commitment to see reality as it *is*. When reality is harsh—as is the case when a loved one dies, for example—then it is actually rational to feel depressed and morose. Pollyannaism, on the other hand, is a refusal to see tragedy even when tragedy exists.

3. Seeking to identify whether one's feelings are based on fact or on distortions does not alter the fact that feelings can be complicated; it simply makes feelings a little easier to handle.

4. Implying that "since life is complicated, one shouldn't be rational" is like saying "since medical school is difficult, nobody should become a doctor" or, "since raising children is difficult, nobody should have kids." The fact that a venture is complicated is all the more reason to adopt a principle by which to master it. And the way to master life is to learn to be rational—where "rational" is understood to mean adherence to the facts, with the help of logic, and enjoying one's emotions on that assumption.

Based on the above, do I have sufficient data to support my emotional conclusion?

My emotional conclusion is based upon a distortion of the concept "rational," as well as a failure to recognize that a general method is required for physical and psychological survival: the method of reason or, more specifically, introspection. Since my emotional conclusion is based upon mistaken assumptions, it is incorrect.

Rational Course(s) of Action/Methods for "Letting Go" of Irrational Conclusion:

1. Replace the socially popular definition of "rational" with the correct one—i.e., listening to and respecting my feelings, but using evidence and logic as the final arbiters in any dispute between my thoughts and feelings.

2. Reinforce the correct definition whenever I experience an automatic negative reaction being rational. Remind myself that feelings need to be listened to but not accepted as facts. To use a courtroom analogy, feelings act as the *testimony* but not as the *verdict*. Only reason and introspection can lead me to a verdict.

3. Learn to develop a positive attitude about placing facts above feelings. Try to counter the conventional wisdom that becoming rational means being repressive or intolerant. Look for evidence to suggest that becoming more rational necessarily leads to uncaring or unfeeling behaviors; what basis is there for such a conclusion? Keep my mind open to the possibility that I might actually turn out to be a calmer, kinder person by using such an approach.

4. Ask myself this question: if I don't use reason as a method of coping with my emotions, what am I to use in its place?

Feeling: "My therapist does not care about me and my problems. He only wants the money."

Facts Which Support This Conclusion:

1. My therapist does expect payment each session.
2. If I forget to pay him, he reminds me to do so.

3. He charges me for sessions that I cancel with fewer than two days' notice.
4. When I hint about how I do not like the price of therapy, he does not offer to lower his price.

Facts Which Support A Different Conclusion(s):

1. My therapist works very hard to help me. He seems interested in helping me solve my problem and sometimes our sessions even go over by a few minutes.
2. When I canceled an appointment and did not reschedule, he left a message for me indicating that he wanted to see how I was doing. He asked that I call him back even if I did not wish to schedule an appointment.
3. He seems to enjoy what he does and takes pride in it.
4. He seems concerned that the therapy be effective. At the end of every session or two, he asks me for feedback regarding how the session went and if either of us, including him, needs to be doing anything differently.

Based on the above, do I have sufficient data to support my emotional conclusion?

Despite my feeling it does not look that way. My feeling says that he *only* cares about money. But the four points on the second list prove that he does care about other things. What I do know for sure is that he cares about being paid. But is this necessarily a problem? Everyone cares about being paid, including me. How would I feel if I did not get paid on my job? Does this mean that I don't care about doing a good job just because I want to be paid? Of course, a therapist is supposed to be a caring, giving person. Is it possible to be a caring, giving person and still accept money for what one does? I have to say yes. I know lots of people that I consider to be caring but who still accept money for what they do.

Rational Course(s) of Action/Methods for "Letting Go" of Irrational Conclusion:

1. Reinforce the facts against the feeling whenever the negative feeling comes up. I have established, beyond any doubt, that my therapist does not care *only* about the money. I can just ignore that feeling in the future, because I have already established it to be false. It will gradually go away on its own, so long as the facts remain the same.

2. Consider bringing this feeling up to the therapist. Perhaps others have done so before, and perhaps he'll have some thoughts about it. So far I've only hinted. Maybe he's even willing to lower his price and I don't know it!

3. Even if he does not lower the price, treat the problem of payment as a positive. It enables me to hold him accountable for doing good work. Imagine if he were not being paid by me, but was being paid by a third party such as the government. He might not feel as pressured to do good work since his income would not depend so directly on being competent. Also, I would not have the power to expect good work of him, since my leaving therapy would not rep-

resent much of a financial loss to him. So even looking at this issue in strictly financial terms, it makes no sense to view the payment as a total negative.

[**Note:** Clearly, the healthy, rational conclusions are not going to come automatically to most individuals. It can take months or even years of effort, including psychotherapy, for an individual to reprogram his ideas to the form described above.]

References

1. Ayn Rand, "The Psychology of Psychologizing," *The Objectivist* (March 1971).
2. Jonathan Rosman, *Freud: Basic Theory and the Philosophies that Influenced Him* (Taped lecture) (Laguna Hills, CA: The Jefferson School of Philosophy, Economics and Psychology, 1991).
3. Leonard Peikoff, "Determinism" in Harry Binswanger, Ed., *The Ayn Rand Lexicon* (Ontario: New American Library, 1896), p. 122.
4. Ayn Rand, "The Stimulus and the Response," in *Philosophy: Who Needs It* (New York, Signet, 1982), pp. 137–161.
5. For a good introduction to the methods of cognitive therapy, see Aaron T. Beck, A. John Rush, Brian F. Shaw and Gary Emery, *Cognitive Therapy of Depression* (New York: The Guilford Press, 1979); also see Aaron T. Beck, *Cognitive Therapy and the Emotional Disorders* (New York: Meridian, 1976). See also, Aaron T. Beck, Gary Emery and Ruth L. Greenberg, *Anxiety Disorders and Phobias: A Cognitive Perspective* (Basic Books, 1985).
6. David Burns, *The Feeling Good Handbook* (New York: Plume, 1989), p. 61.
7. Leonard Peikoff, *Objectivism: The Philosophy of Ayn Rand* (New York: Dutton, 1991), pp. 73–109.
8. John Leo, "Higher Education as Therapy," in *The Washington Times,* May 19, 1994.
9. Stanton Peele, *The Diseasing of America: Addiction Treatment Out of Control* (Boston: Houghton Mifflin Co., 1989), p. 221.

10. Edith Packer, "Understanding the Subconscious," *The Objectivist Forum,* Feb. and April 1985.

11. David Burns, *Feeling Good: The New Mood Therapy* (New York: New American Library, 1980), p. 45.

12. Ayn Rand, "Philosophy: Who Needs It," in *Philosophy: Who Needs It* (New York: Signet, 1982), pp. 5–6.

13. Leonard Peikoff, *Objectivism: The Philosophy of Ayn Rand,* p. 159.

14. *Ibid.,* p. 159–160.

15. Edith Packer, *The Art of Introspection* (Laguna Hills, CA: The Jefferson School of Philosophy, Economics and Psychology, 1985). The techniques of introspection provided in this book are a modified version of an approach developed by Dr. Edith Packer, as described in the above article. While the general principles underlying my method and that of Dr. Packer are the same, the specifics of her six-step approach differs from mine in a number of ways. For example, I emphasize rational courses of action in addition to changing mistaken assumptions as part of the therapeutic exercise. For more information on Dr. Packer's technique of introspection, I refer you to the above article.

16. Ayn Rand, "Philosophical Detection," in *Philosophy: Who Needs It,* pp. 12–22.

17. Aaron Beck, *Cognitive Therapy and the Emotional Disorders,* p. 12.

18. Leonard Peikoff, *Objectivism: The Philosophy of Ayn Rand,* pp. 110–151.

19. Aaron T. Beck, *Cognitive Therapy and the Emotional Disorders,* pp. 47–75 and 245–262.

20. Melody Beattie, *Codependent No More* (New York: Harper & Row, 1987).

21. *Ibid.*, p. 172.
22. Ayn Rand, *Introduction to Objectivist Epistemology* (New York: Meridian, 1967), p. 69.
23. *Codependent No More*, p. 172.
24. *Ibid.*, p. 173.
25. Leonard Peikoff, *Objectivism: The Philosophy of Ayn Rand*, pp. 303–310.
26. Melody Beattie, *Codependent No More*, p. 174.
27. Stanton Peele, *The Diseasing of America: Addiction Treatment Out of Control*, p. 57.
28. *Ibid.*, p. 59.
29. B. S. Tuchfeld, "Spontaneous Remission in Alcoholics," *Journal of Studies on Alcohol*, 42 (1981), pp. 626–41.
30. L. R. H. Drew, "Alcoholism as a Self-Limiting Disease," *Quarterly Journal of Studies on Alcohol*, 29 (1968), pp. 956–67.
31. Stanton Peele, *The Diseasing of America: Addiction Treatment Out of Control*, p. 76.
32. Melody Beattie, *Codependent No More*, pp. 51–55.
33. *Ibid.*, pp. 78–79.
34. *Ibid.*, pp. 89–100.
35. Leonard Peikoff, *The Ominous Parallels* (New York: Stein & Day, 1982). Also, "Contemporary Philosophy: A Report from the Black Hole (Part II)," by Gary Hull, in *The Intellectual Activist*, July 1993.
36. Christina Hoff Sommers, *Who Stole Feminism?* (New York: Simon & Schuster, 1994), p. 43.
37. *Ibid.*, p. 231.
38. *Ibid.*, p. 257.
39. Diana E. H. Russell with Laura Lederer, "Questions We Get Asked Most Often," in *Take Back the Night: Women on Pornography*, ed. Laura Lederer

(New York, William Morrow & Company, Inc., 1980), p. 29.

40. Sandra Lee Bartky, *Femininity and Domination: Studies in the Phenomenology of Oppression* (New York: Routledge, 1990), p. 15.

41. Senate Committee on the Judiciary, *Hearings on S. J. Res. 61 and S. J. Res. 231, Proposing an Amendment to the Constitution of the United States Relative to Equal Rights for Men and Women,* 91st Con., 2nd sess., 1970 (Washington: U.S. Government Printing Office, 1970), p. 155.

42. Carol Gilligan, *In a Different Voice: Psychological Theory and Women's Development* (Cambridge, Mass.: Harvard University Press, 1982), p. 8.

43. Betty Friedan, *The Second Stage* (New York: Summit Books, 1981), p. 229.

44. Colette Dowling, *The Cinderella Complex: Women's Hidden Fear of Independence* (New York: Summit Books, 1981), p. 31.

45. See Margaret Talbot, "Where the Boys Aren't," in *The Washington Post Magazine* (11/20/94), p. 19.

46. Senate Committee on the Judiciary, *Hearings,* p. 4.

47. See Margaret Talbot, "Where the Boys Aren't," p. 17.

48. Nora Johnson, "Housewives and Prom Queens, 25 Years Later," *New York Times Book Review,* 20 March 1988 p. 33.

49. Madeleine L'Engle, "Shake the Universe: A Spiritual Vision," *Ms.,* July/August 1987, pp. 182, 219.

50. M. F. Belenky, B. M. Clinchy, N. R. Goldberger and J. M. Tarule, *Women's Ways of Knowing: The Development of Self, Voice and Mind* (New York: Basic Books, 1987).

51. See Margaret Talbot, "Where the Boys Aren't," p. 19.

52. Susan Haack, "Epistemological Reflections of an Old Feminist," presented at annual meetings of the Eastern division of the American Philosophical Association, Washington, D.C. (December 1992). Sponsored by the Social Philosophy and Policy Center, Bowling Green. Haack's paper was published in *Reason Papers* 18 (Fall 1993): 31–43. This excerpt appeared on p. 33.

53. Carol Gilligan, *In A Different Voice: Psychological Theory and Women's Development.*

54. Andrea Dworkin, *Woman Hating* (New York: E. P. Dutton & Co., Inc., 1974), pp. 20–23.

55. See Margaret Talbot, "Where the Boys Aren't," p. 19.

56. Thomas Sowell, *Inside American Education: The Decline, The Deception, The Dogmas* (New York: The Free Press, 1993), pp. 103–244.

57. Carol Gilligan, *In A Different Voice: Psychological Theory and Women's Development,* pp. 17–18.

58. Barbara Deckard, *The Women's Movement: Political, Socioeconomic, and Psychological Issues* (New York, Evanston, San Francisco, London: Harper & Row, 1975), p. 430.

59. M. Seligman, "Depression and Learned Helplessness," in *The Psychology of Depression: Contemporary Theory and Research,* ed. R. J. Friedman and M. M. Katz. (Washington: Winston-Wiley, 1974), pp. 83–113.

60. Stanton Peele, *The Diseasing of America: Addiction Treatment Out of Control,* pp. 203–229.

61. See Margaret Talbot, "Where the Boys Aren't," p. 35.

62. Lynn Sherr and Jurate Kazickas, *Susan B. Anthony Slept Here* (Times Books, 1994). As reported in *USA Weekend,* 6/24/94. See also, Bruce Wetterau, *The*

New York Public Library Book of Chronologies
(New York: Prentice Hall Press, 1990).

63. Elizabeth Loftus and Katherine Ketcham, *The Myth of Repressed Memory: False Memories and Allegations of Sexual Abuse* (New York: St. Martin's Press, 1994).

64. Jay Haley, *Problem Solving Therapy* (San Francisco: Jossey-Bass, 1976).

65. Stanton Samenow, *Inside the Criminal Mind* (New York: Times Books, 1984).

66. American Psychiatric Association, *Diagnostic and Statistical Manual of Mental Disorders, Fourth Edition* (Washington, D.C.: American Psychiatric Association, 1994).

67. Stanton Peele, *The Diseasing of America: Addiction Treatment Out of Control,* p. 133.

68. Jane Healy, *Endangered Minds: Why Children Don't Think and What We Can Do About It* (New York: Touchstone, 1990), p. 154.

69. Ayn Rand, "The Psychology of Psychologizing" in Leonard Peikoff, ed., *The Voice of Reason* (New York: Meridian, 1989), p. 24.

70. American Psychiatric Association, *Diagnostic and Statistical Manual of Mental Disorders, Fourth Edition* (Washington, D.C., 1994).

71. Jonathan Rosman, M.D., *Freud* taped lecture, The Jefferson School, 1991.

72. Leonard Peikoff, "Subconscious" in Harry Binswanger, ed., *The Ayn Rand Lexicon* (Ontario: New American Library, 1986), p. 484.

73. Jonathan Rosman, M.D., *Freud* taped lecture, The Jefferson School, 1991.

74. *Ibid.*

75. Leonard Peikoff, *Objectivism: The Philosophy of Ayn Rand,* p. 187.
76. Ayn Rand, *Introduction to Objectivist Epistemology,* p. 16.
77. For a more thorough discussion of this philosophical point see Leonard Peikoff, *Objectivism: The Philosophy of Ayn Rand.*
78. B. F. Skinner, *Beyond Freedom and Dignity* (New York: Knopf, 1971).
79. Edwin Locke, "Behaviorism and Psychoanalysis," in *The Objectivist Forum* (February, 1980).
80. James Hillman, *A Blue Fire: Selected Writings by James Hillman* (New York: Harper, 1989).
81. *Ibid.,* p. 18.
82. *Ibid.,* p. 162.
83. *Ibid.,* p. 153.
84. *Ibid.,* pp. 155–156.
85. Leonard Peikoff, *Objectivism: The Philosophy of Ayn Rand,* p. 164.
86. For a more thorough and philosophical discussion of the arbitrary, see Leonard Peikoff, *Objectivism: The Philosophy of Ayn Rand,* pp. 163–171.
87. The Health Security Act of 1994, sponsored by President Bill Clinton and never passed by Congress.
88. For a more detailed, philosophical discussion of the concept of rights, see Ayn Rand, "Man's Rights" in *The Virtue of Selfishness* (New York: Signet, 1961–64), pp. 92–100. Also see Auberon Herbert, *The Right and Wrong of Compulsion by the State* (Indianapolis: Liberty Classics, 1978).
89. See Alan Greenspan, "Antitrust" in *Capitalism: The Unknown Ideal* (New York: Signet, 1946–62), pp. 63–71. See also, Ayn Rand, "Notes on the History

of American Free Enterprise," in *Capitalism: The Unknown Ideal* (New York: Signet, 1946–62), pp. 102–109 and Gerald Gunderson, *The Wealth Creators: An Entrepreneurial History of the United States* (New York: Dutton, 1989).

90. This is precisely what the original Clinton plan (proposed Health Security Act, 1994) sought to do. The plan forbade "the payment of bribes and gratuities to implement the delivery of health services and coverage." Despite what the bill's supporters claimed, this statement would have been interpreted in courts and by government agencies to mean that no voluntary, private contracts could be initiated between doctors and patients. The government, under such a law, would at last control the practice of medicine in its entirety. Although the Clinton plan failed, I believe that this provision will resurface in the future because advocates of national health insurance are determined to realize their goal no matter how long it takes.

91. See George Reisman, "The Real Right to Medical Care Versus Socialized Medicine" excerpted from *Capitalism* (Ottawa, IL: Jameson Books, 1996). Also see: Americans for Free Choice in Medicine, *A Free Market Approach to Health Care Reform* (Newport Beach, CA, 1994) and Edward Annis, *Code Blue: Health Care in Crisis* (Washington, D.C.: Regnery Gateway, 1993).

92. British NHS examples courtesy of Deroy Murdock, New York writer and president of Loud and Clear Communications. His article entitled, "British Health, Not Exactly an Inspiration" appeared in *The Washington Times,* August 19, 1994.

93. Again, the source is my physician/colleague in Canada. I will not provide his identity because he is at the mercy of government officials for his livelihood. The same may someday be true of American health care providers, if medical and mental health care is increasingly regulated and even nationalized.

94. Norman T. Berlinger, "A Mortal Science," in *Discover* (September 1994), pp. 30–35.

95. Ludwig von Mises, *Socialism* (Indianapolis: Liberty Classics, 1981 reprinted edition).

96. Americans for Free Choice in Medicine, 1525 Superior Avenue, Suite 100, Newport Beach, CA 92663, has detailed information on free-market health care reform.

97. David Seabury, *The Art of Selfishness* (New York: Pocket Books, 1937), p. 176.

98. Nathaniel Branden, "Emotions and Repression (Part II)" in *The Objectivist* (September 1966).

99. Stanton Peele, *The Diseasing of America: Addiction Treatment Out of Control,* p. 246.